Eat Clean, Eat Safe

Eat Clean, Eat Safe

Dodging Food Dangers and Learning to Shop for, Prepare and
Love Healthful Meals Anytime, Anywhere You Go!

CLAUDIA DEL VECCHIO, CDN
BARRY M. GREY

ISBN: 1507650981
ISBN 13: 9781507650981
Library of Congress Control Number: 2015901028
CreateSpace Independent Publishing Platform
North Charleston, South Carolina

Dedication

This book is for all who wish to eat and live healthily, which also means *safely*. It's dedicated to Chubbs, our family's beloved pet pug of almost seven years, who died suddenly after eating tainted treats.

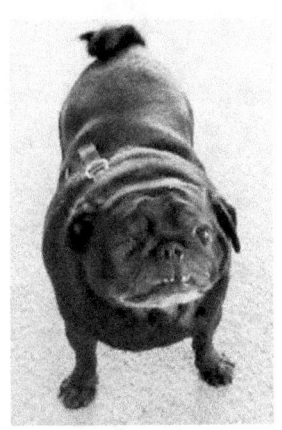

No one should have to lose a loved one—animal or human—to the clearly preventable tragedy of food poisoning.

Sadly, we did not suffer alone; many others have lost cherished pets under similar circumstances.

This book is designed to help protect you and those you love from food poisoning that could be lurking where you least expect it. Knowledge is power and safety.

And in a way, it is love too.

—Claudia Del Vecchio, CDN
Los Angeles, California
April 2015

Table of Contents

Foreword

It may seem glib to employ the metaphor "body politic" in a book about food safety in America. The Renaissance-born term refers to a country's entire populace, usually in contexts involving medicine, politics or both. The metaphor is here because after more than a century of government regulation and enforcement, American bodies remain startlingly at risk due to a failure of political leadership to adequately identify and address critical breaches in the safety of the country's food supply.

There's no question that the Food and Drug Administration maintains strict guidelines and a rigorous focus on medications and supplements. Yet agency efforts aimed at protecting the food supply have not dramatically reduced the number of contamination-based recalls.

There are any number of potential bottom-line reasons for this, including the money-spreading influence of food industry lobbyists on Congress, a perception that consumers have minimal interest or, especially, the shortage of funding or manpower or both to effectively police such a gigantic industry.

On healthy eating habits, there is some progress to report. A long-term study released by the Harvard School of Public Health[1] in 2014 found a modest improvement in adult American eating habits between 1999 and 2010.

---

1 Dong D. Wang, Cindy W. Leung, Yanping Li, Eric L. Ding, Stephanie E. Chiuve, Frank B. Hu, Walter C. Willett, "Trends in Dietary Quality among Adults in the United States, 1999 through 2010," *JAMA Internal Medicine* 174, no. 10 (2014): 1587-95.

But there's an unfortunate flip side to the study. Harvard found a widening healthful-diet gap between wealthy and poor Americans.

Lower-income adults landed below the average, with scores that barely moved over those dozen years. And the statistical gap between well-to-do and less well-off Americans actually increased. Therefore, those with lower incomes (and scores) face comparatively higher risks for obesity, heart disease, strokes and diabetes.

Income levels, of course, mean little if the food supply is equally unsafe for both rich and poor. And at its core, food safety is largely a matter of food quality. Unsafe conditions lead to tainted food, which threatens public health and erodes the increasingly limited government resources available to cover the costs of treatment. What's worse, as you'll soon read, is that some food-borne diseases can produce long-term health issues. Ask anyone whose seemingly routine case of "food poisoning" turned into a serious lifelong disorder whether food safety gets enough attention these days.

The vulnerability of the food supply to contamination poses some enormous challenges. The most obvious involves everyday Americans. With this book, the authors hope to generate a growing consumer awareness of, and demand for, safer and cleaner foods. The public health consequences of shrugging off the problem are almost unthinkable, especially when so many antibiotics now are being outsmarted by the mutating bacteria they're meant to destroy.

A public outcry, of course, requires meeting the next challenge—developing more effective, serious, comprehensive and easy-to-grasp public education on the critical need for clean, safe foods.

And science will be pressed to deliver on the third challenge—that of thoughtful, benign advances in food technology ensuring that safer foods and ingredients are readily available.

Finally and perhaps most importantly, we believe proper, achievable and simple-to-understand new guidelines and standards on consumer food safety are a necessity. They can come from advocacy groups, the food industry or the federal government.

Naturally, we'd prefer teamwork by these various parties; each clearly has a vested interest in seeing clean, healthful, nutritious food become the norm, not the purview of specialty stores. In this age of fractious politics and raging rhetoric, would such cooperation even be possible? We hope so, since the only thing at stake is the health and viability of the American body politic itself.

—Kurt Hong, MD, PhD
Director, Center for Clinical Nutrition and Applied Health Research
Keck School of Medicine of the University of Southern California
Los Angeles, California
April 2015

Introduction

Have you looked at your food lately?
Seriously.

When it comes to what people eat, most assume the best about what's on the plate in front of them. And why not? Who wants to hunker down with an oozing, beefy, melty-cheesy, grilled-onion-laden, hopelessly overstuffed 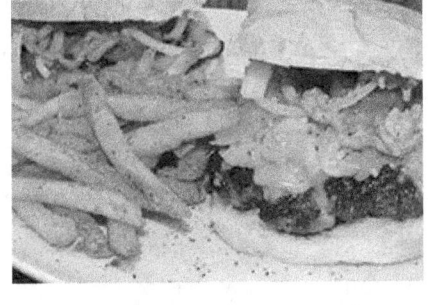 burger—bivouacked with a pile of fries, no less—thinking, "Yeah, I can't *wait* to be doubled over and marooned in the bathroom for the next twenty-four hours."

They dismiss all doubts about the freshness, safety and healthfulness of their meals at home or at any kind of dine-out or takeout venue.

Big mistake, *nos petits gourmands.*

Enough to Make You Sick

Chances are, you already know somebody in your office, at school or on your job site who, when calling in sick, claimed food poisoning. C'mon, didn't you roll your eyes just a little? It always sounds, uh, fishy—especially during great beach weather, or on opening day of the baseball season, or when Katy Perry tickets are going on sale downtown, first come, first served.

Well, if you had doubts over such a telephoned tale of woe, time to reconsider. Think about this:

In 2011, the Centers for Disease Control estimated that one of every six Americans gets sick annually from a food-borne illness. Counting along with us at home? That works out to a staggering *forty-eight million people!*

Every year.

Of those, 128,000 will be hospitalized. And 3,000 will die.

Don't blame the government messenger. Guesstimating illnesses, hospitalizations and deaths is among the CDC's routine responsibilities, a standard but important public health practice.

These guesstimates provide proof of the unpleasant power of pathogens. Here's another shock: Such normally transitory illnesses can and do leave a significant number of people with agonizing, soul-crushing medical complications that devastate them *for life.* That's among the great underreported stories of modern medicine, one we'll address in this book.

Sure, it's easy to dismiss all this. After all, presented by themselves, government statistics are enough to make anybody sick—or bored, anyway.

The fact is, these are pretty grim figures—data you can't just laugh away. You don't have to work the counter at a Vegas sports book to know that with one-in-six odds, you've got a great chance at some point to be really, really sick.

So the natural follow-up question is, "Well, just what am I supposed to do, now that I've been exposed to these nasty little McNumbers?"

Clean Diet, Dirty Secrets?

You hear it all the time: "clean diet."

Go ahead, Google the ubiquitous catch phrase. You'll find "clean diet" has become part of the lexicon. In fact, you know it's caught on when celebrities bring it up in interviews. Unfortunately, it's usually those shining stars who never learned the value of unexpressed thoughts, the ones who call news conferences to tell the world they've stubbed a toe.

Like Gwyneth Paltrow.

She described to *SELF Magazine* in 2013 how the clean diet has affected her relationship with then husband[2] Chris Martin of the band Coldplay: "You feel lighter and your emotions get smoother."

Uh, right. Thanks, Gwynnie.

Now, about clean diets. They're usually described something like this:

"Eat nothing but small meals throughout the day. Limit yourself to unprocessed, whole foods—fruits and veggies, whole grains, lean meat.

"Dump saturated fats, trans fats and overprocessed things like white flour, sugar and sugary sodas. Juices. Anything artificial or containing preservatives.

"And [gulp]…alcohol."

For the record, when the doctor recommended she cut out dairy, sugar, gluten and processed foods, a horrified Gwynnie blurted out, "What the——— am I going to eat now?"

Would it be cruel to suggest crow?

The typical clean diet rules and guidelines—and there are many more— are admirable. But how could anyone truly and successfully follow this regimen over the long haul when there are so many insidious trip wires, roadblocks and dirty little secrets standing in the way?

Like, for example, the previously noted passing parade of popular pathogens.

How safe and healthful can everyday meals be when an estimated forty-eight million Americans a year get food poisoning? Not very.

---

2   During much of 2014, the status of Paltrow and Martin's legal relationship remained unsettled. In the spring, they announced a "conscious uncoupling," followed by months of seesaw news accounts indicating possible reconciliations. It's all too complex for mere mortals to follow or interpret.

Clean Diet: No Paltrovian Panacea

The clean diet and its variations are certainly healthful alternatives to the eating habits of most Americans. But the reality is that most of us eat out regularly—grab-and-go lunches, fast food, fine dining, business dinners, starch cathedrals doubling as dorm cafeterias, coffee-and-muffin meet ups, you name it. And there's just no guarantee that, whatever recipe or venue is involved, restaurant food is necessarily safe.

And at home, people assume their kitchen food-prep habits are, if not entirely proper, at least not dangerous.

Pathogens, however, don't discriminate on the basis of recipe, race, color, sexual orientation or pizza preference; they're equal opportunity illness factories. Stomach issues can be generated by any number of food-borne allergens, microbes and toxins. And pathogens can play a role in weight issues. Studies are underway into the suspected correlation between food-borne illness and subsequent weight gain.

While everyone's at risk and no one's immune from food-borne pathogens, those most susceptible include young children, the elderly and people already suffering from some kind of illness.

We're Here to Help

This book aims to map out, clearly, reasonably and without a lot of needless complexity how to recognize and reduce food-borne risks to your health.

Even better, we'll provide simple information on how to enjoy delicious, healthful meals at home or away—and how to shop for, store and prepare meals that can head off those teeny but powerful stomach-churning varmints at the pass.

One

Outbreaks, Food Recalls and the ABCs of Microbial Miscreants

Our weekend road trip to Vegas is just about done.[3] We've checked out of our posh, five-star hotel/casino on the Strip. But before hitting the highway to LA, we stop for a bite at the hotel café.

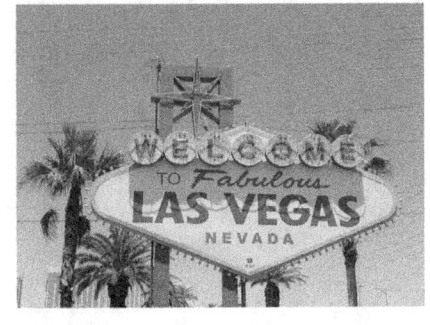

This coffee shop lets us watch the meals being prepared. Ordering a tuna sub, we're relieved to see the cook is wearing gloves. But the relief is brief because she plops the bread slices of our developing sandwich onto the tabletop—smack in the middle of various meat juices, food particles, mystery stains and more that hasn't been cleaned up.

There's no sign of the parchment paper that chefs are supposed to lay down to ensure food doesn't get contaminated. We complain—politely, but loudly, too. But she keeps on going, seemingly on autopilot and with the sole response, "I know, I know. It's coming. It's coming."

---

3 A true story. Really! It happened to Claudia.

We flag down a manager and describe what's happening. "All employees are trained in food safety," she responds helpfully, "and that employee knows better."

Gee, thanks. If the food worker knows better, why doesn't she follow basic, legally mandated food-safety guidelines? How often do you think this happens? And more importantly, what happens to us *after* we consume tainted meals?

These two questions are at the heart of why this book was written.

Well, you've probably guessed we leave without ever touching the sandwich. Next stop: just down Las Vegas Boulevard, to yet another five-star hotel/casino on the Strip. This time it's pizza, again made right before our eyes.

A slice of cheese pizza, we think. *They can't screw this up*. And we're in luck—it's so busy that the manager is working the floor, this being Football Sunday.

We're getting hungry and also impatient to get on the road. When at last they call our number, we stride purposefully to pick up the presumably germ-free pizza. "Here you go," the manager says, handing off the slice like the quarterback on the nearby TV monitor handing off the football. And with the confidence of a running back spiking the ball after a touchdown, he slaps the receipt right atop the cheese.

Where it sticks. *Yuck!*

Isn't *this* manager trained in food safety? Doesn't *he* know better? Is this a conspiracy by a cabal of Nevada gastroenterologists?

In less than an hour, we find ourselves *twice* placed in direct jeopardy of contracting any number of the food-related ailments often lumped together under the umbrella of "food poisoning." The Vegas-style odds are high, every day, that we're all susceptible to becoming ill in this fashion—through no fault of our own.

Driving home, we begin mentally composing the screenplay for a promising movie sequel: *Leaving Las Vegas 2: Doubling Down While Doubled Over*.[4]

---

4 We resisted the temptation to call the sequel *Heaving Las Vegas 2*. You're welcome.

Is this tale needlessly ominous? Do we overstate our case? We really don't think so, even if life often seems to have devolved to an endless parade of warnings—some dire, some dumb.

The more benign caveats include things like radio traffic reports, movie and TV disclaimers ("No aardvarks were teased in the making of this film") and the classics from childhood:

"Wait an hour after eating before getting back in the pool, or you'll get cramps."

"Brush after every meal, or your teeth will fall out."

And everybody's favorite: "It's all fun and games until somebody loses an eye."

Sure, your parents' hysterical warnings never rang true; deep down, even adult Chicken Littles know this. But plenty of everyday alerts count—like cancer warnings on cigarette packs, nutrition labels on packaged food and auto-recall notices.

Familiarity breeds contempt—or maybe just indifference. Perhaps that's why people tune out the near-constant stream of warnings about compromised food that crop up daily across the spectrum of American gastronomic life.

Some might assume that with a trusty, efficient, savvy government on the job, poisonous food would be a vague, distant memory, like phone booths, VCRs and Murphy beds.

After all, it's not unreasonable to think poisoned food was relegated long ago to the bus tray of history. Really, the food industry should have cleaned up its act as far back as 1906. That's when Upton Sinclair's shocking, fact-based novel *The Jungle* exposed filthy, indecent, real-life conditions in American meatpacking. The landmark book quickly inspired federal legislation creating both the Food and Drug Administration and government oversight of meat inspection. A half century later, the feds extended inspection to poultry. And by law, state inspections must be as rigorous as federal standards.

So, problem solved, right? Not so fast, omnivore.

Devastating Complications

Every time you turn around, the stakes involved in food-borne illness go up. According to various studies, the damage done by some bacteria extends far beyond temporary ailments like diarrhea and vomiting or nasty, recurring disorders such as urinary tract infections in women. Food poisoning outbreaks have been linked to long-term, life-changing, sometimes life-threatening complications. In fact, experts believe serious, chronic complications may occur in 2 to 3 percent of food-borne illness patients. Let's look at four complications that can make "temporary tummy trouble" a frightening misnomer.

HEMOLYTIC UREMIC SYNDROME (HUS)

The main bacterial culprit here is usually *E. coli* but sometimes shigella. Their toxins migrate to the bloodstream to kill red blood cells, which normally carry oxygen throughout the body and shepherd carbon dioxide to your lungs to be exhaled.

Most HUS patients recover, but only after long hospital stays. As much as 5 percent of American HUS patients die, with kids among the most vulnerable.

But perhaps a third of all HUS patients suffer long-term complications. If we forego a lot of unpronounceable, Latin-derived medical terms, these complications can include the following:

- Devastation to the body's production (via bone marrow) of red blood cells meant to replace those lost to HUS
- Blood platelet deficiency. And when you lose platelets, your blood stops clotting. And when your blood stops clotting, minor nicks and cuts don't stop bleeding. And when you can't stop bleeding...
- The inability to eliminate human waste, which builds up, turns poisonous and can produce cognitive breakdowns including psychosis, seizures and coma
- Serious, life-threatening heart ailments

- Pancreatitis, or inflammation of the organ producing enzymes for digestion and hormones to regulate the body's use of sugar. Symptoms range from medium to severe pain in the upper abdomen and sometimes the back. Sometimes chronic pancreatitis develops after just a single attack.
- Acute respiratory distress syndrome, something as bad as it sounds
- Kidney damage and kidney failure

GUILLAIN-BARRÉ SYNDROME (GBS)

Campylobacter[5] is the main culprit behind this crippling disorder disrupting the body's peripheral nervous system—those nerves and associated cells outside the spinal cord that wire the central nervous system to the arms and legs. GBS occurs after the immune system goes haywire from the presence of foreign pathogens. GBS can cause varying degrees of paralysis and can be life-threatening if it attacks the respiratory muscles, thus shutting down your ability to breathe.

REACTIVE ARTHRITIS, A.K.A. REITER'S SYNDROME

Often traced to the infections salmonella, *E. coli*, shigella and campylobacter, this food poisoning complication develops when the well-intentioned immune system releases otherwise heroic antigens into the bloodstream to attack invading bacteria from tainted food. The unintended result is serious joint inflammation and other arthritis-like conditions, particularly in the knees and joints of the ankles and feet. Other targets include the eyes, skin and urethra.

For most patients, reactive arthritis symptoms come and go, usually disappearing for good within a year. But until then, you could be in a world of hurt.

---

5 Campylobacter is also among the underlying causes of ulcerative colitis. Similar to the notorious Crohn's disease, ulcerative colitis is a chronic, painful inflammation of the rectum and the lining of the large intestine. You really don't want this—trust us.

Post-Infectious Irritable Bowel Syndrome (IBS)

If you've endured IBS, or know someone who has, you're already aware that this chronic, often long-term disorder is as painful, disruptive and embarrassing as anything you can get from exposure to bacterially contaminated food or water. According to the International Foundation for Functional Gastrointestinal Disorders,[6] IBS shows up in about 10 percent of those who've *already recovered* from the dirty work of the usual suspects—*E. coli*, salmonella, shigella, campylobacter and norovirus.

Symptoms can show up at regular intervals or unpredictably, often turning routine social situations into anxiety-riddled public adventures. IBS's symptoms include diarrhea, constipation, bloating and abdominal pain. Patients also get saddled with a "racing to the restroom" urgency and—there's no polite way to put this—mucus in the stool.

◆ ◆ ◆

So despite a myriad of health, food inspection and safety laws, many contaminants continue to compromise the food supply, big time. And, to be fair, slaughterhouse conditions aren't always to blame; mistakes or mechanical failures involving refrigeration can also nurture bacterial threats. Regardless, this is where so many modern warnings, alerts and notifications come in. Or as they're known in government, the food industry and the media—*recalls*.

The Not-So-Magnificent Seven

In general, food-related recalls and public warnings involve four main pathogens plus three health-hostile issues. The pathogens include listeria, *E. coli*, salmonella and bovine spongiform encephalopathy, better known as mad cow disease. The three additional issues are antibiotic resistance, food expiration dates and a category we simply call Weird Stuff in Food We Just Couldn't Make Up.

In this chapter, we'll cover the first four, each qualifying as a microbial monster.

---

6   Just imagine what their annual conventions are like.

LISTERIA

It's neither a germ-killing mouthwash nor a West African republic known for enormous oil tankers.[7] Actually, *Listeria monocytogenes* is a potentially fatal bacterium found in soil, water and animals. This dangerous little mercenary puffs out his chest, plants his flag in your lunch and proceeds to infect you with the food poisoning listeriosis. It's one nasty, often mysterious sucker that spreads via the body's natural interstate highway system, the bloodstream.

Those infected with listeriosis might not show the symptoms—high fever, severe headache, stiffness, nausea, abdominal pain and diarrhea—until weeks after exposure. By then, the sufferer likely is hospitalized, and the odds of identifying the suspect meal or dish aren't much better than those of finding a specific grain of sand on Santa Monica beach. While blindfolded. In a downpour.

The CDC identifies listeriosis as the third most common cause of death from food poisoning, killing about 320, or about *one of every five,* of the 1,600 Americans it sickens every year. Ninety percent of victims are those least equipped to fight it off—pregnant women, their fetuses and newborns (the pathogen can cause miscarriage and meningitis), the elderly and those with already-compromised immune systems.

Another worry: listeria can grow in cold temperatures. So unlike the gelatinous villain in *The Blob,*[8] which recoiled from the cold, listeria actually *thrives* in chilly climates.

There are hundreds of listeria-linked recalls each year, both voluntary and government-mandated. And listeria is an equal opportunity pathogen, forcing regional and nationwide recalls affecting huge conglomerates and smaller-scale food suppliers alike. Some of the biggest fast-food franchises also were hit with food-related recalls.

If numbers tell us anything, it's that no matter how careful you are, practically no one is really safe from listeria infection—federal safety standards or not—because nobody can truly control how most food is grown or raised, processed, prepared, preserved or transported.

---

7 Listerine and Liberia, respectively.

8 The 1958 teen-oriented hit starring Steve (billed as "Steven") McQueen in his first starring role, with Aneta Corsaut, later Andy Griffith's TV love interest, as McQueen's girlfriend.

Chew on this:

In 2011, America's deadliest listeria outbreak in nearly ninety years killed at least 33 Americans and sickened another 147. The culprit: infected cantaloupe grown in Colorado.

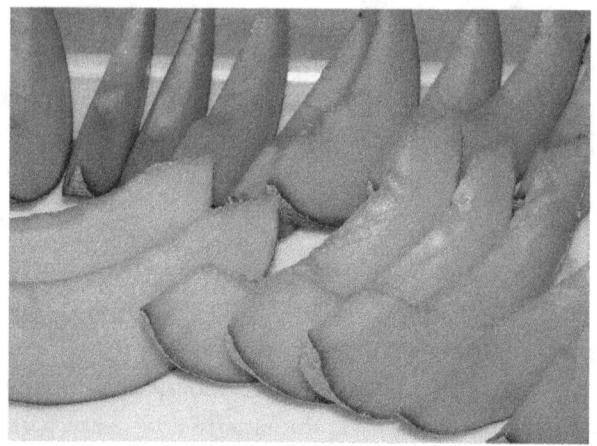

Yes, a sweetly innocent melon, the humble cantaloupe.

Investigators concluded the twenty-eight-state outbreak may have been the result of a contaminated potato-washing machine, dirty water on the floor of the growers' packing center or both.

Here's a classic example of how consumers remain powerless to foresee or evade many food-borne dangers—proof that the strictest rules and regulations in the world can't always prevent disaster.

In recent years, listeria—a highly ambitious bug of evil intent—has planted his little flag of disease in foods including raw sprouts, raw (unpasteurized) milk, cold deli meats, uncooked hot dogs, soft cheeses, smoked fish and precut celery (in chicken salad). It tainted other vegetables including cilantro, spinach and onions, stir-fry veggie combinations, various salads and slaws.

But wait, *there's more!* Other contaminated foods included dips, salsas, cakes, mushrooms, frozen chicken dinners, fajita mixes, steak toppings, cheesesteak sandwiches, meatballs, both chicken and beef patties and—cue a triumphantly ironic fanfare—even packets of sliced apples promoted as healthful menu choices by McDonald's and Burger King.

E. COLI

Does *E. coli* have a better publicist (or these days, "brand manager") than other pathogens? You'd think so—*Escherichia coli* does seem to get a lot more press than, say, listeria. Maybe it's the mystique of using a first initial. Like J. Edgar Hoover or G. Gordon Liddy.[9]

Whatever the reason, *E. coli* is considered among the worst *E. vil*–doers in the pathogen cosmos. If you've thought, "Gosh, I don't even *remember* hearing about *E. coli* before 1982," you're one canny citizen. The bug wasn't identified until that year, during an outbreak of hemorrhagic colitis. And the *E. coli* bandwagon didn't really get rolling until 1993, when a multistate megaoutbreak was linked to undercooked meat patties sold by a major fast-food chain.

These days, the CDC reports nearly 73,500 confirmed *E. coli* infections a year. And that's just the tip of the microbe. The *actual* number clearly is much higher, since so many people tough it out without bothering to tell their doctors or public health agencies.

Technically, *E. coli* is not a single bacterium but a clan of six hateful critters. The most common villain on the family's North American side is *E. coli* O157:H7. After exposure, diarrhea and cramps usually turn up within two to eight days; other strains bring urinary tract infections, respiratory illness, bloodstream infections and kidney failure (in extreme cases) and have been linked to diabetes, high blood pressure, heart disease and stroke.

Several strains are sweetly benign, vacationing amiably in your intestinal tract. But pathogenic, or dangerous, variants of *E. coli* also enjoy setting up shop in the intestines of humans and animals, plus in water too. Some strains are also spread by simple person-to-person contact.

Most *E. coli* sufferers recover on their own, often within a week, although severe cases produce harsher symptoms that hang on much longer.

The majority of *E. coli* O157:H57-related infections involve meat. A typical recall, in July 2013, involved fifty thousand pounds of suspect ground meats—beef, chuck and sirloin. The meat products were recalled nationwide

---

9 Or F. Scott Fitzgerald, H. Ross Perot, H. Norman Schwarzkopf, C. Everett Koop, A. Bartlett Giamatti, E. Howard Hunt, J. Paul Getty, L. Ron Hubbard, M. Night Shyamalan, S. Epatha Merkerson, F. Lee Bailey, J. Walter Thompson, L. Frank Baum and W. Somerset Maugham.

from retailers, wholesalers and food-service distributors by National Beef Packing Co. of Kansas. Just a month earlier, the same firm yanked back nearly twenty-three thousand pounds of ground beef for the same reason.

Beyond ground beef not cooked internally to at least 160 degrees Fahrenheit,[10] you're most likely to be infected with *E. coli* by consuming many of the same edibles that spread listeria—raw (unpasteurized) milk and juice, raw fruits and veggies (especially those pesky alfalfa sprouts) and raw cheeses, that is, those made from raw milk.

Packaged vegetables pose another risk. In November 2013, more than ninety tons of ready-to-eat salads and sandwiches were recalled due to *E. coli*. Twenty-six people in three states became sick after eating the tainted foods sold by a Northern California catering company to various major grocery retailers.

(An encouraging 2014 study out of Washington State University suggested a surprisingly simple breakthrough in preventing the spread of *E. coli*. Details on that in chapter 10.)

Drinking or swimming in contaminated water also puts you at risk of catching *E. coli*. And watch out for petting zoos or any place you can reach out and touch farm animals including cows, sheep and goats. Make sure you wash your hands immediately and thoroughly after direct contact.

SALMONELLA

Contrary to legend, salmonella is not a story about a beautiful fish forced to dress in rags and scrub the sea bottom while her nasty stepsisters attend a fancy ball at the Sands.

Salmonella is no fairy tale. It's a very real, potentially deadly set of related bacteria causing the infection salmonellosis, marked by (see a trend here?) diarrhea, abdominal cramps and fever lasting up to a week following an incubation period of twelve to seventy-two hours. Most cases resolve themselves, but extreme salmonella infections can spread from the intestines to the bloodstream to the far reaches of the body.

The CDC reports about four hundred deaths each year among the forty-two thousand reported cases of salmonellosis. Again, the key word here is

---

10   More on proper cooking temperatures near the end of this chapter.

reported because the CDC notes the number of unreported cases (milder or undiagnosed) is thought to be as much as *thirty times higher!* That's roughly 1.26 million annual cases of salmonellosis. So you can see just how devastating an all-out bacterial epidemic could be.

Proving its cruel streak, salmonella preys on the young by infecting creatures (such as those at petting zoos) that kids are drawn to, including pet turtles, baby chicks or ducklings, small rodents and reptiles.

The many salmonella-related recalls in recent years provide a typical list of the kinds of foods in which this "sociopathogen" enjoys hiding. Just a few of those recalled foods: smoked salmon, eggs, mangos and "tuna scrape"—a yellowfin tuna product made of back meat scraped off fish bones, producing bits of tuna with a ground-up appearance.

As with other pathogens, those most vulnerable to salmonella include the elderly, people with already-compromised immune systems and young children. In one horrifying instance, a seven-year-old Australian girl contracted a severe case of salmonella poisoning after eating a chicken wrap at a KFC location in Sydney. She suffered serious, permanent brain damage and is confined to a wheelchair. In April 2012, a court ordered KFC to pay her family $8.3 million, according to a CBS/AP news report. KFC Australia vowed to appeal.

Mad Cow

Few food-borne outbreaks have captured the fearful imagination of a vulnerable public like bovine spongiform encephalopathy (BSE), otherwise known as mad cow disease. Although a frequent pop-culture punchline, there's nothing funny about BSE, a progressive, fatal neurological disorder 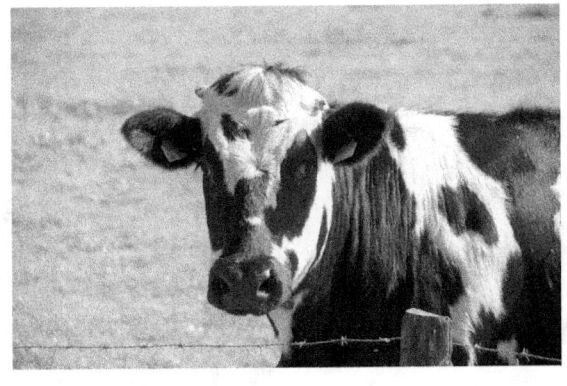 in cattle. If you've seen the notoriously heartbreaking footage of delirious cattle falling over dead from BSE, you know it's nothing to laugh at, especially since an animal's physical and mental descent typically extends over a period of thirty months to eight years. During that time, mad cow disease slowly turns healthy cattle brains and spinal cords to spongy mush.

What's this got to do with you? Just that mad cow is most easily transmitted to humans who consume foods containing contaminated cattle brains, spinal cord or digestive-tract tissue.

No small bit of mystery surrounds the infectious agent that transmits BSE. It's a "misfolded" (i.e., mutant) protein called a prion. When passed to humans, the disorder is known as Creutzfeldt-Jakob disease. As of October 2009, it had killed 166 people in the United Kingdom—the worst-affected country—and 44 other people around the world.

How did all this happen? Scientists point to a rather grotesque, short-sighted practice by some ranchers, namely that cattle, which are herbivores by nature (i.e., veggie and salad buffs), were themselves infected when fed the ground-up remains of meat and bone meal from their brethren cattle.

You don't hear much about mad cow lately. But despite eradication efforts, it's still lurking. In 2012, the Agriculture Department's confirmation that a California dairy cow tested positive set off a nationwide panic in the US beef community.

A Review for You

In a world rife with hysterical warnings, some recalls glide past our consciousness simply because we become inured to them. That's likely the case with many recalls and warnings each year about tainted food and its potential for disease—fleeting, long-term or life threatening.

In this chapter, we've discussed four food contaminants that routinely threaten human health and safety and that are among the microbial world's most troublesome A-list pathogens:

- **Listeria.** A potentially fatal bacterium found in water, soil and animals, this bug's symptoms—high fever, severe headache, stiffness, nausea, abdominal pain and diarrhea—can take weeks to develop. Listeria is especially hostile to pregnant women, the elderly and people with compromised immune systems, and it haunts a wide variety of foods.

- **Salmonella.** This potentially deadly family of bacteria causes the infection salmonellosis. After an incubation period of three days, the symptoms—diarrhea, abdominal cramps and fever lasting up to a week—often resolve themselves. But don't get comfortable; about four hundred US deaths are attributed each year to salmonellosis, and the actual number of infections easily could be thirty times higher than the official government figure of forty-two thousand.

- *E. coli.* Among six related bacteria in the *E. coli* family, the most common "coli cousin" in North America is *E. coli* O157:H7. It produces diarrhea and cramps within two to eight days; other strains bring urinary tract infections, respiratory illness, bloodstream infections, kidney failure (in extreme cases) and other disorders. Most often found in improperly cooked meat, *E. coli* also hides out in raw milk and cheese, fruits and vegetables, especially alfalfa sprouts.

- **Bovine spongiform encephalopathy** (BSE, otherwise known as mad cow disease). Thought to be the result of cattle being fed ground-up, infected brain and spinal cord tissue of other cattle, BSE kills beast and human alike.

"What You Can Do" Checklist: Shopping without Dropping

It's easy to be intimidated by all the potential perils out there, including myriad microbes and other sources of food poisoning we haven't even mentioned. But with a little knowledge and common sense, you too can laugh in the face of pathogens and other such *E. vil*–doers. Here are the first of some quick-reference food safety checklists we're including at the end of selected chapters.

Food Shopping Safety Guidelines

The first line of food defense for you and your family is at the grocery store. Being supermarket savvy about produce, dairy, meats and seafood can greatly reduce the odds of food-borne illness. The following tips are based on information from the Academy of Nutrition and Dietetics, WebMD.com, the US Department of Agriculture Food Safety and Inspection Service and the San Diego County Department of Environmental Health.

METHOD TO YOUR SHOPPING MADNESS

- ✓ Know your source! Shop only in reputable grocery stores, farmers' markets or restaurants. And don't buy food from an unpermitted street vendor—no one-dollar taco is worth two weeks of misery.
- ✓ Begin your store visit by shopping first for nonperishables, such as paper products, canned or boxed foods, etc. Don't buy cans with bulges or dents on any seams. Check boxed or packaged foods for signs of insects or rodents. Check expiration dates on all infant formula or foods.
- ✓ Next, head for frozen foods. Check for signs of thawing—ice crystals on the packaging, softness in the food item or discoloration of the product. Don't buy a product unless it's completely frozen.
- ✓ Pick up your refrigerated items last. Wrap raw meats in a plastic bag and place on the shelf beneath the cart. Never stack raw meat atop ready-to-eat foods, produce or any can or bottle you may drink from.
- ✓ Make the deli counter and dairy cases among your last stops before checkout. Place deli meats beside other cold items in your grocery cart so they can share the chill and the thrill of freshness. Check manufacturers' "use by" dates on lunch meats and don't buy beyond those periods.
- ✓ Reusable grocery bags are all the rage, now that the outright ban (or discourage-by-taxation) movement is spreading like a fast-food-fed waistline. But while this is good for the planet, the movement poses an unanticipated health risk. If the reusable totes, often made of

canvas, aren't laundered regularly, bacteria from food packages tend to hang around. A 2012 study determined that the norovirus assault on a girls' soccer team in Oregon was due to tainted totes. Best practice: use separate totes for raw meats and poultry, and machine launder the bags after each use. Also, resist the convenience of stashing totes in the car trunk because that often-humid environment can be a breeding ground for microbial miscreants.

PICK PRODUCE PRUDENTLY

- ✓ Enjoy shopping at farmers' markets? Go early in the day—you'll snag the freshest items and avoid produce that baked in the heat all day.
- ✓ At the supermarket, buy individual produce items, not the prepackaged vegetables (such as bags of salad or four-to-a-pack green peppers), so you'll have more control over what you bring home.
- ✓ If you see produce bearing any hint of mold, bruises or cuts, walk on by, as the song says.
- ✓ Only purchase what your household will use within a week.
- ✓ Only buy pasteurized juices; things like unpasteurized apple cider can't always be trusted.

CHECK DAIRY AND UDDER MILK PRODUCTS

- ✓ Check those telltale "sell by" dates on all dairy products.
- ✓ Only buy eggs in cartons that are cold; whenever possible, confirm the eggs aren't cracked or broken.

FISH FOR SEAFOOD SAFETY

- ✓ Especially with fish, buy only from trustworthy sources, like grocery stores and specialty seafood markets.

- ✓ Make sure fresh fish is properly refrigerated, appears shiny and firm and isn't separating from the bone. If it smells fishy instead of fresh and mild, cast your line elsewhere.
- ✓ Packaged seafood should be displayed in ice, with packages tightly sealed and free of dents and tears. Skip those packages with ice crystals inside—this means the seafood previously thawed.
- ✓ Buy unwrapped, cooked seafood (shrimp, crab, smoked fish, etc.) only if it's in a separate case from raw fish because bacteria can make the leap and contaminate the cooked cousins.

MEAT YOU CAN EAT, AND HOW TO MINIMIZE THE SULTRY IN YOUR POULTRY

- ✓ Check to see packaging is tightly sealed and very cold to the touch.
- ✓ Buy only packaged chicken appearing pink, not gray.
- ✓ If a package has passed the "sell by" date, pass it up for one still within its freshness window.
- ✓ On packages of bacon and fresh sausage, always look for the Safe Food Handling label, which both affirms the meat has undergone proper processing and includes handling and cooking tips.
- ✓ Get meat and poultry bagged separately from other groceries; leakage of natural juices could infect other things you're buying.

Common Sense in the Kitchen

When you return from the supermarket, keep your family safer by remembering some simple rules.

JUST CHILL ALREADY

- ✓ Use a refrigerator thermometer to confirm the temperature inside is at or below forty degrees Fahrenheit.

✓ Place frozen items in the freezer immediately; immediately refrigerate food requiring refrigeration. Maintain potentially hazardous foods (PHFs) such as meats, dairy products and other items at that same forty degrees Fahrenheit.

✓ Don't overload the fridge! Make sure there's enough space inside for cold air to circulate and chill everything properly.

You Can't Be Too Clean

✓ Wash hands and clean and sanitize cutting boards, utensils, countertops and all food-contact surfaces, including the kitchen sink. Do all this before beginning food preparation and between prep steps, when contamination can make an unwanted comeback.

✓ Use soap and hot water to clean surfaces and bleach to sanitize them. Your sanitizing solution should be a teaspoon of bleach per quart of water. Use portable plastic cutting boards that can be washed and sanitized in a dishwasher.

✓ Don't use sponges to clean dishes or other food-contact surfaces—they're the kitchen equivalent of bacterial condos. And let dishes air-dry, either in the drainer or dishwasher, before putting them away.

More than a TV Show

By law, food preparation professionals must follow the "20/20" rule and you should too:

✓ At least every twenty minutes, scrub your hands with liquid soap (from a pump bottle) and hot water for at least twenty seconds.

✓ Dry your hands with disposable towels before handling food, immediately after using the restroom, between tasks such as handling raw chicken or making a salad, or any other time necessary to prevent food contamination.

A Separate Peace

- ✓ Keep raw meat, poultry and seafood separate from ready-to-eat foods.
- ✓ Likewise, separate raw foods from cooked foods.
- ✓ Store raw meats in the fridge beneath ready-to-eat foods such as salad, fruits or leftovers.
- ✓ Place raw meats in containers so their natural juices don't drip onto and risk contaminating other stuff.
- ✓ Rotate food products by using the rule of FIFO—"first in, first out"—to ensure food is not left long enough in the fridge to spoil.

We Thaw What You Did

- ✓ Keep frozen food continuously frozen—don't refreeze anything unless you've *gone ahead and cooked it first.*
- ✓ Thaw food products in any of the following ways: in the refrigerator, under cold running water, in a microwave oven or as part of the cooking process.

Now You're Cookin'

- ✓ Use an accurate food thermometer to ensure you're cooking to the following safe internal temperatures:

  - ○ 145°F for whole meats, allowing the meat to "rest" for three minutes before carving or consuming. This will ensure the juices remain in the meat, not dripping out of it, when you begin slicing.
  - ○ 160°F for ground meats.
  - ○ 165°F for all poultry.
  - ○ 165°F for reheated foods. Reheat rapidly by heating small portions on the stove or in the microwave.

DEFENDER OF THE FAMILY

✓ Be especially careful when preparing food for children, pregnant women, people in poor health and older adults—remember that listeria and salmonella consider them target markets.

✓ Wash all fresh fruits and vegetables thoroughly before storing, preparing, cooking or eating.

✓ Don't cook when sick, especially if you have diarrhea or have been vomiting.

✓ Rat out those bacterial interlopers—report suspected food-borne illnesses to your local health department. You could be a hero by stopping an outbreak in its tracks.

✓ Store leftover foods in containers with tight-sealing lids to avoid contamination; you'll definitely be a hero, at least to Tupperware party hosts.

WHAT, MORE WARNINGS?

✓ Avoid eating food products with raw (unpasteurized) eggs such as homemade cookie dough, cake or brownie batter. They are great—until you're doubled over with food-borne illness.

✓ Use pasteurized egg products in recipes traditionally made with raw eggs—such as Caesar salad dressing, hollandaise sauce, homemade eggnog or shakes with raw eggs.

YOU *CAN* HANDLE THE TRUTH

✓ Use tongs or other tools for handling food whenever possible.

✓ Never handle food or utensils if you have open sores or cuts on your hands. If you must handle food, use food service gloves to protect you and your family.

Keep Those Vermin Squirmin'

- ✓ Keep doors closed and make sure window screens fit snugly.
- ✓ Remove trash promptly from food preparation areas.
- ✓ Trash containers should be leak proof and covered.
- ✓ Be sure plastic trash bags are securely tied off before placing in dumpsters or other refuse containers.
- ✓ Check all food or packaging for signs of insects, staining, mouse droppings, mold growth, damaged containers, offensive odors or other signs of contamination or spoilage.

Two

Fighting the Resistance, Weird Stuff and the *Real* Meaning of All Those Expiration Dates

In chapter 1, we introduced you to the four most patently pathological pathogens inhabiting the world of food-borne illness. We follow up in chapter 2 with three additional issues facing the safety of the food supply. They aren't really microbial threats to human health, but we find discussing them to be, uh, *irresistible*.

Antibiotic Resistance

Remember at the end of *Casablanca* when Bogie and Claude Rains decide to join the Resistance and fight for the good guys? You wouldn't see that ending today—not if today's Resistance movement was backing psychotic, evil microbial malcontents resistant to modern antibiotics. (Yeah, this is a stretch. Stay with us.)

Consider a warning from the medical community that you've heard for years:

Don't use antibiotics unless absolutely necessary, lest humankind's microbial enemies become resistant to them, leaving you vulnerable to current and future bacterial threats.

They're not kidding. Here's what happens:

When bacteria are exposed to an antibiotic, they begin adapting—that is, figuring out ways to get around a medicine's effectiveness. This happens in both humans and animals and in the general environment. Once the bacteria wise up, they multiply, spread quickly, infect their hosts and generously tip off other bacteria about how they did it. Thus, other germs learn to thumb their little noses at hapless hosts, too.

"Each time bacteria learn to outsmart an antibiotic," the Centers for Disease Control declares, "treatment options are more limited, and these infections pose a greater risk to human health."

The CDC calls human resistance to antibiotics a "quickly growing, extremely dangerous problem" and cites international concern that such "nightmare bacteria" pose a "catastrophic threat" to people across the earth.

Tough rhetoric, but numbers back it up. According to the CDC, at least *two million people* become infected with resistant bacteria each year, and among those, twenty-three thousand die. Many more perish from complications of such antibiotic-resistant infections.

Exposure to these armor-clad bacteria is as simple as inhaling the breeze as you walk down the street. The CDC reports that most infections occur in the community, often in healthcare settings but also via sexually transmitted diseases and skin infections. Among the most prominent is MRSA, a potentially fatal form of *Staphylococcus aureus* resistant to antibiotic medications usually prescribed for ordinary staph infections.

But what about infected livestock that, through overexposure to antibiotics before slaughter and shipment to market, face the same risk of defenselessness? The sad, daunting fact is that food animals "serve as a reservoir of resistant pathogens and resistance mechanisms that can directly or indirectly result in antibiotic resistant infections in humans," according to the CDC.

One strategy to consider is avoiding factory-farmed meats and adopting a more plant-based diet.

It's important to note, however, that while antibiotic resistance remains a widely accepted threat, some medical experts don't believe it's irreversible. One school of thought maintains people can undo the resistance simply by staying away from antibiotics for extended periods so that the body can naturally rebuild its immune defenses. Given the split of opinion in the medical establishment, perhaps the common sense solution is to err on the side of caution and keep your intake of antibiotic medications to an absolute minimum. It also means avoiding, whenever possible, factory-farmed meats and dairy foods produced with the use of antibiotics.

Weird Stuff in Food We Just Couldn't Make Up

If you neutralized all the pathogens threatening the human food supply, there'd be little need for this book, right? Yet thanks to human error, year after year the strangest things turn up in turnips, fall into falafel and inhabit ice cream. So as a public service, here's a quick survey of true yet quite surreal meals.

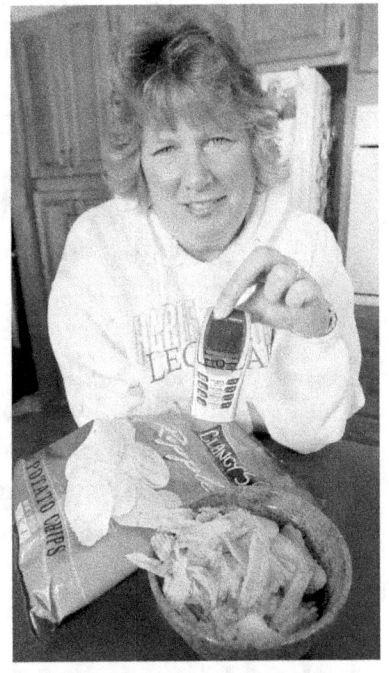

In 2009, snackin' Emma Schweiger of Janesville Township, Wisconsin, was enjoying some Clancy's Potato Chips when the bag produced a bigger than bite-sized surprise: a Nokia cellphone. She told the Janesville *Gazette* that the gadget, covered with a greasy potato chip film, didn't work. No word on whether it was hampered by a defective chip—Intel or otherwise.

A carbs-lovin' lassie in Northern Ireland got more fiber than usual early in 2010. The BBC reported that while chewing a slice of Hovis brand whole wheat bread, she discovered part of a very hairy-looking oven mitt. She found the rest of

**Snackin' Emma Schweiger
photo by Dan Lassiter /
courtesy Janesville Gazette**

the glove baked inside the remainder of the loaf. The baking company involved was fined £750.

The lounges at Applebee's Neighborhood Bar and Grill deserve a hipper rep, considering all the lizards that keep turning up. In 2003 in Coralville, Iowa, as the Associated Press reported, a lizard head was found in a carryout salad from the local Applebee's. The head tested negative for salmonella. Five years later and one state over, in Bloomington, Illinois, a dead, four-inch lizard was found intact, again in an Applebee's salad. No indications that either lounge lizard was wearing a silk suit.

And according to various news accounts, other surprises turning up in restaurant meals in recent years included the following:

- Syringes in a fast-food hamburger
- A mouse in fried chicken from a major chain
- A dead frog inside a can of big-name soda
- Part of a thumb in a fast-food-chain sandwich, traced without difficulty to the restaurant manager, whose thumb was bandaged
- Human unmentionables in ice cream served up as retaliation at an Australian restaurant, where the staff evidently didn't appreciate the customer's attitude
- A black widow spider ("She mates and she kills"[11]) that came gratis with grapes purchased at a California health foods supermarket
- A condom in a bowl of clam chowder served at a high-end seafood restaurant in Irvine, California
- A seven-inch blade baked into the bun of a sandwich served at a big-name sandwich shop in Queens, New York

Admittedly, some of the grotesque stories above could make you ill just thinking about them. We don't mean to frighten—although fear *is* considered a great motivator by hiring managers and political consultants—but to underscore that no matter how many food safety laws are on the books, human error, inadequate procedures and sometimes plain old malice can make any meal—fancy or fast, at home or on the town—an exercise in dining roulette.

What's important is to use common sense and to follow universally accepted strategies to minimize the danger to your life and health—and, of course, to make mealtime something to be savored, not feared.

---

11 Promotional "tagline" for *Black Widow*, director Brian De Palma's 1987 film thriller with Theresa Russell and Debra Winger.

Expired Food

Expiration dates on food are among the most ubiquitous warnings in everyday life. But did you know most expiration dates and comparable warning dates are purely voluntary? In fact, the only federal mandates for expiration dates involve infant formula and some baby foods. (Some states, however, demand dairy products be pulled from shelves on their expiration dates.) Unfortunately, the simplicity of the concept has gotten lost in the startling proliferation of terminology turning up on food packaging. Here's a quick primer on what they really mean:

- **"Expiration" date.** The last, final, ultimate, no-kidding, drop-dead date a food should be eaten or used by.
- **"Sell by" date.** Actually intended for the retailer, this instructs shelf stockers how long something should remain on display. It doesn't necessarily mean a food is unsafe after that date. Still nervous? Ease your mind— don't buy anything past the "sell by" date. And don't be embarrassed to reach past the older items in front, like milk cartons, to snag a fresher package at the back  of the refrigerated case. No one will think less of you.
- **"Best if used by" date.** This refers only to flavor or quality, not safety.
- **"Born on" date.** This refers to the specific date of manufacture. You'll see this most often on beer, in which nasty microorganisms can appear and multiply after three months.
- **"Guaranteed fresh" date.** This pops up most often on bakery items, which are edible after the date, although not at their freshest.
- **"Use by" date.** The manufacturer's recommended last date for peak quality.

    Manufacturers pick these dates. Rhetorical question of the day: are they passively suggesting you toss out still-edible products and buy replacements earlier than you'd expected? To pad their bottom lines? Just sayin'.

- **"Pack" date.** This tricky one usually is found on canned or packaged goods—but often in a super-secret code to tease your feverish brain. The protocol could be an easy-to-grasp month-day-year convention (MMDDYY) or, if the manufacturer is sadistic, an obscure alpha-numeric system only decipherable by nuclear weapons engineers and teenaged millionaire app designers.

A Review for You

This chapter provided a thumbnail sketch of a few issues affecting food safety, including the following:

- The increasing threat of antibiotic-resistant bacteria in food, a looming worldwide problem traced to the overprescribing of medications for bacterial infections.
- Weird Stuff in Food We Just Couldn't Make Up, our mostly-for-fun category highlighting humanity's innate gift for inventive gross-outs. From cell phones to vermin and from bandages to condoms, the mere existence of Weird Stuff is a salute to creative contamination.
- The food industry's head-spinning collection of expiration and warning labels that demand simple explanations.

"What You Can Do" Checklist: Drug-Resistant Infections and More

Here are some easy and simple ways to prevent the creation or spread of drug resistance:

- ✓ When you're sick, don't automatically demand antibiotics from your doctor and don't take antibiotics not prescribed for your specific illness. When meds are properly prescribed, don't skip doses; follow explicitly the doc's dosage and duration directions.

✓ Get updated and regular vaccinations against drug-resistant bacteria.

✓ Wash your hands before eating or after visiting the bathroom.

✓ Wash those very same hands after handling uncooked food; you don't want to ingest drug-resistant bacteria that live on that raw food, do you?

✓ Carefully follow temperature and cooking instructions to kill resistant bacteria in meat and poultry.

✓ Keep in mind there is some disagreement in the medical community about antibiotics, with some experts believing a person's resistance can be stopped or reversed simply by going cold turkey and not taking antibiotics for long periods of time.

✓ Eat organic. Organic milk, eggs and meat aren't exposed to the drugs during production, so they contain fewer antibiotic-resistant bacterial strains.

How Long Is This Good For?

Here are a few suggestions for how long popular proteins are safe in the refrigerator (not freezer) after purchase:

✓ Poultry	1 or 2 days
✓ Beef, veal, pork and lamb	3 to 5 days
✓ Ground meat and ground poultry	1 or 2 days
✓ Fresh variety meats (liver, tongue, brain, kidneys, heart, chitterlings)	1 or 2 days
✓ Cook-before-eating cured ham	5 to 7 days

Three

So far, we've seen that among myriad threats to the food supply, four major ones involve microbial mayhem—five if you count antibiotic resistance, in which diabolical, mutating microvillains self-restore their evil powers before eyeing you as target practice.

Here in chapter 3, we'll present some general info about food-borne pathogens from the Centers for Disease Control and Prevention. And we'll demystify the top five most widespread bugs, describing simply how they do what they do to you—and what they're capable of.

Tip of the Microbial Iceberg

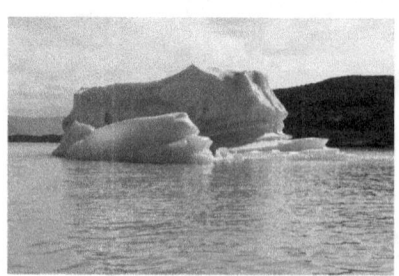

If you thrive on terror but don't feel like waiting for the next entry in the *Saw* movie franchise, check this out:

Remember we mentioned earlier that roughly forty-eight million Americans were sickened in 2011 by tainted food? Thirty-one known pathogens accounted for 20 percent of those illnesses. The remaining 80 percent of cases—representing more than thirty-eight million people—were caused by *mystery toxins*, which the CDC euphemistically calls "unspecified agents." Bottom line: four of every five American victims of food-borne illness *probably never knew what hit them!*

So who (or more properly, what) are these mystery agents? Some remain anonymous because there just isn't enough data to identify them. According to the CDC, others include "known agents not yet identified as causing food-borne illness; microbes, chemicals or other substances known to be in food whose ability to cause illness is unproven; and agents not yet identified."

If you can get past all the known-vs.-unknown pathogen numbers, some other figures are pretty revealing. Those 20 percent of illnesses—the ones caused by the *known* pathogens—accounted for 44 percent of food-related deaths (1,351 in raw figures) and hospitalizations (55,961) in 2011.

Those mystery ("unspecified") agents are blamed for the remaining 56 percent of deaths (1,686) and hospitalizations (71,878).

The numbers practically beg you to take every reasonable precaution against becoming a statistic yourself.

The top-five pathogens contributing to food-borne illness in the United States are the following. (Drum roll, please.)

Norovirus, a.k.a. "the Stomach Flu"

This bug holds the dubious honor of being the national champion of food-borne illness. Each year, norovirus sickens about *twenty million people*—nearly half of all victims of food-borne disease. The highly contagious norovirus is easy to pick up—from an infected person or contaminated food, water or surfaces. And unlike the one-and-done measles, the norovirus family boasts many variations and, as the years pass, is magnanimous enough to nail you again and again.

As many as seventy-one thousand norovirus sufferers are hospitalized each year and up to eight hundred people, mostly older adults, die from it. Insular gatherings are notably vulnerable to noro. In January 2014, about eight hundred vacationers and staff aboard two Caribbean cruise liners fell victim to norovirus. The liners, from different cruise operators, were forced to cut their trips short.

Often called "the stomach flu," noro's not influenza at all. Nor, strictly speaking, is it food poisoning. Rather, according to CDC epidemiologist Dr. Aron Hall, noro is a highly contagious virus that rudely barges into your stomach without asking, usually between November and April, and proceeds to inflame your stomach or intestines with acute gastroenteritis.

And as nasty as the word "gastroenteritis" sounds, the symptoms are even worse: severe diarrhea and vomiting, stomach pain, nausea and sometimes fever. Most recover within three days, although young children and older adults are more vulnerable and sometimes need hospitalization.

Noro spreads easily, in part because when symptoms go away, the virus still can be passed along for another three days. And a noro casualty has billions of virus particles to share with colleagues, friends and family. So beware of getting too close to somebody with the virus—their infectious noro nanobugs can easily flit right into your mouth.

It's just as risky a path to noro-blivion to eat contaminated food, or touch tainted surfaces, and then put your fingers in your mouth. Which can make a fried chicken dinner finger-lickin' dangerous. Don't tell the colonel.

Salmonella: Nobody's Undersea Stepsister

Remember salmonella from chapter 1? Our gal Sal, number two among sources of food-borne illness, is a bacterium of bad intent offering free cases of diarrhea, fever and abdominal cramps (technically called salmonellosis) lasting up to a week.

Sal is a sun worshiper, preferring to spread her bad self in the summer when bacteria more easily contaminate food. She's no food snob, either, getting into a wide variety of noshables starting with eggs and undercooked poultry, then branching out to ground meat, fruits, vegetables and even processed foods like frozen pot pies, among many others.

Speaking of eggs, back in the day a big source of salmonella contamination involved chicken feces that clung to egg outer shells. Regulators thought they'd handled the problem by stepping up standards for cleaning and inspecting eggs.

Alas, the all-clear was short-lived. A certain strain of sneaky salmonella began turning up *inside* the intact shells of Grade A eggs, regardless of outer cleanliness—an illusion worthy of Houdini or David Copperfield until you know the secret:

First, salmonella infects the ovaries of healthy-looking hens, contaminating the inside of eggs *even before the shells are formed.* Which addresses the age-old conundrum, "What came first, the chicken or the egg?" Clearly, neither. It was Sal.

Mystery solved.

Unfortunately, however, the spread of salmonella via poultry remains just as threatening as ever. In early December 2013, the US Department of Agriculture unveiled new plans to fight the pathogen after a very nasty salmonella outbreak was traced to three Foster Farms processing plants in central California. More than four hundred people nationwide were sickened by the especially virulent strain that, according to various accounts published by the *Los Angeles Times*, showed signs of resistance to antibiotics. The US Department of Agriculture suspended operations at one of the plants over what it called "egregious" unsanitary conditions including an infestation of cockroaches.

Let's put some human faces on this outbreak. One is Rick Schiller, a fifty-one-year-old executive who spent five days in the hospital with severe vomiting, diarrhea and an infection that made his joints throb, turned his right leg purple and inflated it to twice its normal size. "I've been around the block," the California ad man said. "I've had some painful things. But nothing like this." Tests linked his salmonella strain, a common one called Heidelberg, to the Foster Farms outbreak.

But Schiller got off easy compared to eighteen-month-old Noah Craten of Arizona, who came down with the same Heidelberg strain from the Foster Farms fiasco. Noah endured a relentless fever for nearly a month before doctors found that a blood infection had caused abscesses on his brain. Surgeons ended up cutting open a piece of his skull to excise them. The toddler spent three weeks in a hospital isolation room before he could finally go home in November 2013.

A few weeks after the Foster Farms chicken outbreak came another foul shock: potentially harmful bacteria were found on 97 percent of raw chicken breasts (of various brands) purchased in stores across the United States. About half were contaminated with at least one kind of bacteria resistant to three or more classes of antibiotics. And about 11 percent of the chicken breasts had two or more types of multiresistant bacteria.[12]

The USDA's Food Safety and Inspection Service called for developing stronger sampling and testing—and creating the first-ever national standards to measure salmonella contamination in cut-up chickens. The agency's under-secretary called it the most comprehensive plan of its kind ever.

The nonprofit Center for Science in the Public Interest, however, was not impressed, quickly calling the plan inadequate and insisting the USDA wasn't addressing a worsening antibiotic resistance associated with salmonella. The group blamed the resistance on drugs used on farm animals to promote growth or prevent disease.

So apparently there's no end in sight for public concern and controversy over salmonella.

CLOSTRIDIUM PERFRINGENS: NEWS, WEATHER AND SPORES

This common spore-forming bacterium (*C. perfringens* to friends), third on our hit parade, kneecaps nearly a million Americans each year, typically delivering diarrhea and abdominal cramps within eight to twelve hours of exposure. But *C. perfringens* does have a heart, sparing victims the fever and vomiting of its contaminant rivals and refusing to be passed from person to person.

C. perfringens has other ways of getting around. It routinely finds environmental hosts that include decaying vegetation, marine sediment, soil and even insects. And it ingratiates itself with precooked edibles and poorly prepared

---

12 "The High Cost of Cheap Chicken: 97% of the Breasts We Tested Harbored Bacteria That Could Make You Sick. Learn How to Protect Yourself," *Consumer Reports*, Feb. 2014, http://www. consumerreports.org/cro/magazine/2014/02/the-high-cost-of-cheap-chicken/index.htm.

foods including meat, poultry and gravies—all this before taking refuge in the intestines of unsuspecting humans and other vertebrates.

Surprisingly, *C. perfringens* at first enjoys such a benign, almost suburban life in an intestinal tract that we've commissioned a sitcom pilot script: *Hangin' with Mr. Perf.* The fun ends when you eat something containing large numbers of *C. perf*.'s fast-duplicating spores. That's when the newcomers join the squatters to produce enough toxin in the intestines to make you sick.

Don't look for any help from heat, either. It may kill hostile invaders in the movies, but in real life, heat just makes *C. perfringens* giggle. For example, in the 1954 sci-fi classic *Them!*, gigantic, nuclear-mutated praying mantises overrun Los Angeles—until the otherwise hapless humans turn flamethrowers on them. But *C. perfringens* spores do just fine in high temps. In fact, when food is held at temperatures between 54 and 140 degrees Fahrenheit, the spores gleefully germinate, prompting out-of-control bacterial growth, especially between 109 and 117 degrees Fahrenheit. The CDC strongly advises reheating any foods held in those conditions before they're consumed.

CAMPYLOBACTER SPP.: WITH CAMPY YOU GET CRAMPY

No, Campy Lobacter isn't a shortstop for the Cubs. Actually, this spiral-shaped bug is a pluralist—he has various permutations, which together provide a generous source of diarrheal illness. But Campy's not all bad; the good news is that not everyone exposed to him gets symptoms.

However, for most people there's bad news: within five days of exposure, campylobacter produces (sometimes bloody) diarrhea, cramping, abdominal pain, fever and occasional nausea and vomiting.

Wait, more good news! Most people recover in two to five days without any specific treatment, assuming they drink extra fluids during their dog days of diarrhea. Antimicrobial meds are only prescribed for severe cases or those at higher risk because of weakened immune systems.

Alas, more bad news: while there are about forty-two thousand confirmed cases annually, or fourteen people diagnosed for every one hundred thousand Americans, a far larger number—the vast majority of cases, in fact—go undiagnosed or unreported. The CDC believes more than 1.3 million people actually come down with campylobacteriosis each year. Worse, campy has a seriously mean streak, occasionally sneaking into the bloodstream to kill patients with those faulty immune systems. Campylobacter infections are thought to kill more than seventy people a year.

On the other hand, the good news is that long-term consequences are rare.

Darn the luck, more bad news: sometimes there *are* long-term consequences—like arthritis and in rare cases, Guillain-Barré syndrome, which tricks the immune system into attacking the body's nerves, producing paralysis (see chapter 1).

On the other hand, campylobacter generally breaks camp in about a week. And that's good news, right?

STAPHYLOCOCCUS AUREUS: THE NOSE KNOWS

Staphylococcus. You're thinking, "That guy on ABC News?" George Stephanopoulos probably gets that all the time. But we sincerely hope he doesn't get staphylococcal food poisoning, the gastrointestinal bug produced by this bacterium. And it's pretty easy to pick up, too—as much as 25 percent of otherwise healthy people and animals have it on their skin or up their noses.

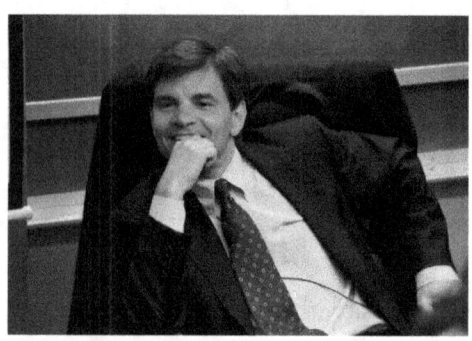

George Stephanopoulos / photo courtesy Tulane University

This industrious illness inspirer conjures up seven different toxins associated with food poisoning. *Staphylococcus aureus* usually spreads to edibles either by contact with food workers or via contaminated milk and cheese. Luckily it's not contagious, so person-to-person exposure is nothing to worry about.

The toxins thrive in salt and salty foods, such as ham. And as with *C. perfringens*, they're impervious to heat, so you can't kill them by cooking.

Staphylococcus aureus pops up most often in unheated handmade foods such as sliced meat, puddings and some pastries and sandwiches.

The fast-acting bug packs a powerful punch of nausea, vomiting, stomach cramps and diarrhea, sending these messengers your way in as little as a half hour—although symptoms more typically appear within six hours of a contaminated meal. Toxin tests to diagnose it are common but not usually administered unless there's an outbreak, often involving contaminated restaurant food. Most cases run their course within three days.

And forget antibiotics. They're useless in the grip of staph's Seven Toxins of Terror. And the CDC reports that staphylococcal toxins are so badass, they actually could be used in a bioterrorist attack.

A Review for You

In this chapter, we found that among the forty-eight million Americans hit with food-borne illness in a typical year (in this case, 2011), four out of five cases involve "unspecified agents"—microbes, chemicals or other substances found in food and believed (research is ongoing) to be contributory.

We then looked at the top-five causes of food-borne illness: norovirus, salmonella, *Clostridium perfringens*, *Campylobacter spp.* and *Staphylococcus aureus.*

- The biggest offender, noro, whacks twenty million people a year and is easily passed along by contaminated people, food, water and surfaces. While it delivers gastroenteritis for about three days, it's really the gift that keeps on giving—you can get it again and again.
- Salmonella strikes most often in summer heat and infects many different kinds of food, but especially poultry and eggs. And because of continuing public health emergencies involving salmonella, in late 2013 the USDA announced it would seek stricter salmonella-detection measures. The program, however, was immediately criticized by some as ignoring the growing threat of Sal's antibiotic resistance.
- *C. perfringens* is the bacterium in a hurry, with spores typically delivering a punishing combination of diarrhea and cramps within eight to twelve hours. And you can't cook it to death; *C. perf.* loves heat. Once

it settles in your intestines, you'll be cooked yourself—but usually for only twenty-four hours.

- Unlike basketball great Campy Russell and baseball's Bert "Campy" Campaneris, *Campylobacter spp.* is a lousy sport. The CDC believes campy cases are wildly underreported and that, in fact, more than a million people a year are knocked flat by this bug. It arrives five days after exposure and takes off in another two to five days. Campy kills more than seventy people a year.
- Political types insist President Nixon had a staph infection.[13] Just shows that pundits are lousy spellers. *Staphylococcus aureus* can produce seven equally unpleasant toxins that can double you up within a half hour (although six hours is more common) and last three days.

"What You Can Do" Checklist: Preventing the Top Five from Deep-Sixing You

KEEP CLEAN AND HEALTHY

- ✓ Wash your hands often with soap and water. If that's not possible, try a hand sanitizer—especially before you prepare food and eat food and after visiting the toilet or changing diapers. Alcohol-based hand sanitizers have their limits, as they don't kill all types of germs (such as norovirus, for example) and are less effective than old-school soap and water—but they're better than nothing.
- ✓ Don't cook or care for others if you're sick, especially if you work in health care facilities, schools or daycare or if you work with food. Wait until your symptoms are two to three days gone before resuming routines in any of these settings.
- ✓ Don't work with food if you've got infections of either the eyes or nose; ditto if there are wounds or skin infections on your hands or wrists.

---

13 Some wags considered H. R. "Bob" Haldeman and John Erlichman to have been Mr. Nixon's chief *staff* infections.

✓ Be extra careful preparing meals for kids, pregnant women, people in poor health and older adults.

✓ Don't drink unpasteurized milk or untreated surface water.

✓ If someone has diarrhea or vomits, quickly clean exposed surfaces and disinfect them with a bleach solution.

✓ To prevent the spread of infection, insist everybody suffering from diarrhea, kids in particular, wash hands with soap carefully and often.

✓ Remove and wash clothes and linens soiled with vomit or feces. Wear rubber gloves and wash your hands after touching these items. Wash clothes and linens with detergent for the maximum cycle length, then tumble dry. (And *don't* put colors in a hot-water load; you *know* they'll fade fast.)

✓ Love your pets? No problem—just don't spread the love unnecessarily. Wash your hands with soap after any contact with, ahem, pet feces. (Do we really need to tell you this?)

PREPARING IT RIGHT

✓ We want this on the record: segregation is a very bad thing. *Except* when it comes to food. Keep raw hunks of protein—meat, poultry and seafood—separate from ready-to-eat foods.

✓ Wash your hands with soap before prepping food, after handling any food that started in this world as an animal and before touching anything else.

✓ Use separate cutting boards for foods of animal origin and those foods that never breathed. Thoroughly clean all surfaces and utensils with soap and hot water after working with the once-upon-a-time animal. Separation prevents cross-contamination.

✓ Rinse fruits and veggies before using or eating them.

✓ Clean surfaces, cutting boards, and counters, then disinfect them with a bleach solution.

Cooking to Kill Germs, Not Guests

- ✓ Prepare beef, poultry, gravies and foods at recommended temperatures—before maintaining them either warmer than 140 degrees Fahrenheit or cooler than 41 degrees Fahrenheit. This prevents the growth of spores that might have survived the cooking process.
- ✓ Cook poultry thoroughly, so it's no longer pink and the juices run clear. This means a minimum internal temp of 165 degrees Fahrenheit. (If a restaurant serves you undercooked poultry, don't be shy—send it back for more heat. But be nice about it.)
- ✓ Serve meat hot, immediately, right out of the oven. Or the covered barbeque. Or grill / griddle / convection oven. Or the microwave oven. Don't forget the skillet / toaster oven / stew pot / hibachi / wok / George Foreman Grill© ("As seen on TV"), or for that matter, any obscure cooking gadget that mesmerized you on an infomercial.
- ✓ Cook shellfish (oysters, for example) thoroughly and to 140 degrees Fahrenheit or higher. Norovirus can survive low cooking temps and even the heat of a quick steaming.

Make It Cool, Reheat It Right

- ✓ Always ensure cold foods are kept cold.
- ✓ Immediately refrigerate leftovers at 40 degrees Fahrenheit or below, or within two hours of preparation. And it's perfectly fine to put hot foods straight into the fridge.
- ✓ If you're outdoors in temperatures 90 degrees Fahrenheit or hotter, safely stash those leftovers in chilly coolers within an hour after the picnic.
- ✓ Large quantities of food—big roasts, whole poultry, potfuls of stew or soup—should be divvied up into smaller portions for refrigeration. Store cooked food in wide, shallow containers and get them in the fridge as quickly as possible.

✓ Cover foods before refrigeration to retain moisture and prevent the smells of some foods from penetrating others.
✓ Reheat leftovers to at least 165 degrees Fahrenheit.

Beware: food may look, smell and taste perfectly fine and still be contaminated, especially if it was left out too long or not prepared properly. So let's be careful out there.

Four

Pet Food Perils and How to Prevent Them

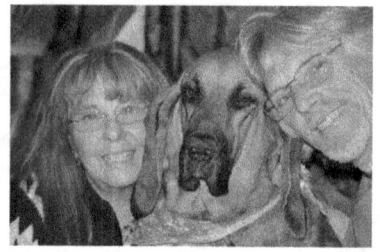

Would you take a bullet for your Bowser? It's not really a trivial question, considering the ferocious devotion animal lovers show their pets. In raising the question, we recall an interview years ago in which Antonio Banderas, speaking of his then four-year-old daughter, told E! Entertainment, "I'd take a bullet for my baby." We know he meant it because he repeated the promise. Twice.

This merits a mention because many pet owners

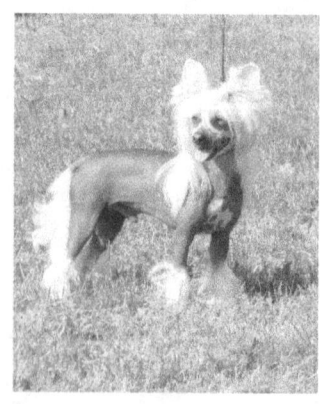

feel as passionately about their furry charges as parents do about their kids. Some even regard pets *as their children*. If they won't take a bullet for Bowser or lie down on the freeway for Fifi, they just might invest in Kevlar body armor, set up road flares, call for an EMT and comfort their little darling during the high-speed ride to the nearest veterinary ER.

The point is simply this: Devoted pet lovers want and need to know how to deal with, and in many circumstances prevent, food-borne threats to their four-legged loved ones.

Beware the Ides of March: Perils in Pet Food

March 15—the notorious "Ides of March." It's traditionally a very bad news day—ask Julius Caesar. Let's recall Shakespeare's take on the events of March 15, 44 BC, when Caesar was assassinated. Knifed by his "friends," the incredulous, dying Roman emperor turned to coconspirator Brutus and asked, "Et tu [you, too], Brute?"

Flash forward to 1917. Three hundred years of Romanov rule ended on March 15 when Russian czar Nicholas II abdicated "in order to save Russia." But Nick saved neither Russia nor his own family. Months later, they were all executed by Bolshevik revolutionaries in the newly christened Soviet Union.

And finally, on the Ides in 2007, the Food and Drug Administration—which regulates food for an estimated 177 million dogs, cats and horses—confirmed widespread suspicions that something was sickening and sometimes killing American cats and dogs: the canned ("wet") and dry ("kibble") food served to Americans' four-legged family members.

In fact, pet poisonings causing kidney failure were popping up worldwide, with cases and associated recalls in Europe and South Africa and across North America. The full extent of casualties—illnesses and deaths—will never be definitively established. The reason was simple—and frustrating. While the FDA heard about eight-five hundred pet deaths, the agency could only positively confirm *fourteen* deaths because of the lack of organized database recordkeeping. On their own, veterinary organizations reported one hundred deaths among more than five hundred cases of kidney failure involving dogs and cats.

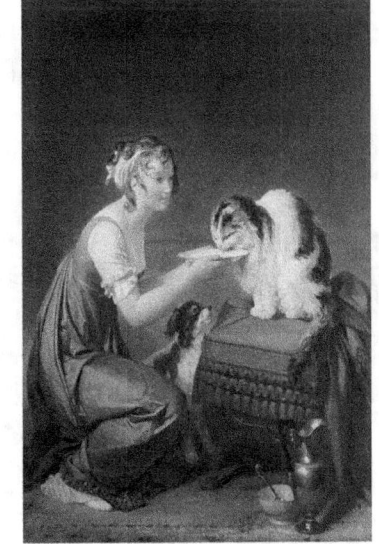

The FDA traced the toxins to Chinese products imported to the United States for use as wheat-gluten filling for pet food. Seems it was contaminated with melamine, an organic compound often mixed with formaldehyde to create a fire-resistant substance used in manufacturing whiteboards, floor tiles, kitchenware, fire-retardant fabrics and other products.

Had this been a good thing, you would've seen pet food commercials boasting of products containing "all the polymer resin a healthy dog needs." But no such commercials exist, not even on YouTube.

The fur flew further. Officials revealed some of the tainted pet food had been used to feed both farm animals and fish. In turn, animals feasting on the bad feed were themselves slaughtered and processed for human consumption.

This represents an ideal example of the theory of transitivity you may remember from grade school arithmetic: If A equals B, and B equals C, then A must equal C.

Let's extrapolate. If tainted feed is consumed by livestock, and those animals then are slaughtered and consumed by humans, then those human diners might also be at deadly risk. Seems intuitive, although back in 2007, government scientists reassured Americans there was little health risk from the tainted feed.

We sure hope they're right.

Was the Great Pet Food Scare of 2007 a fluke? Sadly, no. By late 2013, a mysterious six-year outbreak of illnesses tied to jerky pet treats made in China had killed nearly six hundred pets, mostly dogs, and sickened more than thirty-six hundred others.

The FDA's Center for Veterinary Medicine tested for contaminants but couldn't crack the case.

The extent of problem pet food is further borne out by this: In just six months of 2013—from March through August—the FDA issued health advisories on no fewer than *fifteen* different pet foods. This included wet and dry big-name brands, frozen specialty foods and treat recalls.

Four of the recalls cited possible salmonella contamination, demonstrating old Sal remains an equal opportunity threat to both humans and pets. By

September of 2007, sixty-two people across eighteen states had become ill from the particular salmonella strain called Schwarzengrund.

Fortunately, no one died. All the cases involved contact with dry pet food produced at a single facility, the Mars Petcare US plant in Pennsylvania. (Some were indirect cases of transmission involving human contact with pets that had eaten the Mars Petcare dry food. The company subsequently recalled two of its dry dog food varieties—Red Flannel Large Breed Adult Formula and Krasdale Gravy.)

Significantly, among those people sickened, *nearly 40 percent were just a year old or younger.* Since infants proved especially vulnerable to the infection, parents should take extra care in handling and storing dry pet food, should be vigilant about hand-washing practices, should limit kids' exposure to dry pet food and should be especially selective about where inside the home pets are fed.

Pet food recalls, voluntary or government mandated, continue to be a fact of life in the United States. In the one-year period ending in February 2015, there were no fewer than seventy recalls, with many top-selling brands making the list.[14]

The Rise of Raw

One alternative to commercial product is found in the controversial raw pet food movement. Purely for informational purposes, we present an overview of the movement here—but please note that *in no way do we advocate for, approve of or accept any claims by raw pet food adherents.*

According to WebMD.com, the raw movement began in 1993 when Australian veterinarian Ian Billinghurst, decrying commercial dog food as unhealthy, declared that mature dogs would thrive on an evolutionary diet replicating what canines craved in the days before domestication. (We should note, however, that raw dog food was nothing new at the time, having long been fed to racing greyhounds and sled dogs.)

---

14 "Animal Food Recalls and Alerts," American Veterinary Medical Association, accessed March 12, 2015, https://www.avma.org/News/Issues/recalls-alerts/Pages/pet-food-safety-365-day.aspx.

Billinghurst described his raw rationale with the unfortunate acronym BARF, short for either "Bones and Raw Food" or "Biologically Appropriate Raw Food."

Typical raw dog diets have evolved over time and, according to WebMD. com, now usually contain many of the following:

- Muscle meat, often still on the bone
- Bones, either whole or ground
- Organ meats, including livers and kidneys
- Raw eggs (especially for dogs named Rocky Balboa)
- Vegetables including broccoli, spinach and celery
- Apples or other fruit
- Some dairy, such as yogurt

What, no kitchen sink?

The Raw Repast: No Pet Food Panacea

Regardless of praises sung by raw boosters, there's plenty of notable and credible opposition to raw pet food. Opponents include Lisa M. Freeman, DVM, nutrition professor at the Cummings School of Veterinary Medicine at Tufts University. Freeman's evaluation of raw diets, published in 2001 in the *Journal of the American Veterinary Association*, pointed to online myths and scare tactics about commercial pet food, likely presented and used by backers of raw diets. And citing raw's unbalanced nutritional content, Freeman also challenged purported benefits such as a shinier coat, claiming it's merely the result of high fat levels—something that can actually endanger a pet's long-term health.[15]

There's also criticism of *homemade* raw pet food. Joseph Wakshlag, an assistant professor of clinical nutrition at Cornell University's College of Veterinary Medicine, maintains that such homemade diets can lead to bone fractures and dental problems due to insufficient levels of calcium and phosphorous. (It

---

15   Lisa M. Freeman, Kathryn E. Michel, "Nutritional Analysis of Five Types of Raw Food Diets," *Journal of the American Veterinary Medical Association* 218, no. 5 (2001): 705-709.

should be noted that Wakshlag reportedly accepts some research funding from commercial pet food giant Nestlé Purina PetCare, according to WebMD.com.)

For its part, after a ten-month study by the FDA's Center for Veterinary Medicine (CVM) completed in 2012, the FDA minced neither words nor meat in flatly rejecting raw pet food as a viable alternative to commercial. The study examined 196 commercially available raw dog and cat products, most sold frozen and made from ground meat or sausage.

The analysis went far beyond the issue of nutritional balance: The FDA reported fifteen products (or 7.5 percent) were found smothered in salmonella and a whopping thirty-two raw varieties (16.3 percent) littered with listeria. By comparison, 860 other samples of conventional pet foods and treats, such as semimoist dog food and the like, had exactly *zero readings* for either bacterium. No mention of *E. coli*, either. The sole exception was dry cat food, which recorded a single positive test for salmonella.

Our Raw Recommendation: Just Say Nay

Because of the risk of bacterial exposure posed by raw, the CVM concluded, "the single best thing you can do to prevent infection is to not feed your pet a raw diet." We completely agree. Emphatically. Unequivocally. There's no reason to place your pet in direct dining danger with a risky raw food regimen.

What If Little Schnookims Gets Sick?

Look, if you really named your pet Schnookims, Sweetlips, or anything similarly saccharine, your little loved one is doomed to die of raw embarrassment anyway. But assuming you haven't fatally humiliated little Muffy, if you note obvious symptoms of distress—vomiting, diarrhea, lethargy and so on—then promptly contact the proper authorities.

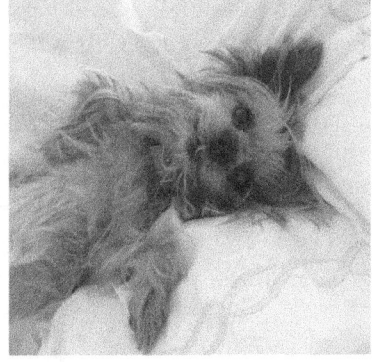

And just who would they be? Federal health officials track and tackle food safety issues affecting both animals and humans. There are two ways to report suspect pet food. First is via the Safety Reporting Portal, an interagency governmental web page hosted by the Department of Health and Human Services. It's easy to use and easy to find if you do a web search for "Safety Reporting Portal."

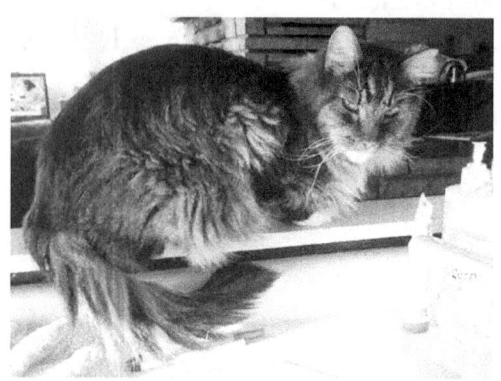

photo by Nancy Schalk

The other route is to telephone the FDA Consumer Coordinator in your state. Just search online for "FDA Consumer Coordinator" and follow links to the page with appropriate telephone numbers for every state.

When you report dry pet food problems, the feds will need important information printed on the packaging—the exact variety, the manufacturing plant and the production date. So when you get home from the store, don't transfer dry pet food into other containers; retain the original packaging until all the food has been safely eaten. The authorities will also want to learn about any overt problems with the product—whether it gave off a foul odor or looked off-color, whether the pouch (or, in the case of wet food, can) was bulging, swollen or leaking, and whether any foreign object was found inside. Other questions will involve the following:

- The exact name of the product and its description from the product label
- The type of container—that is, box, bag, can, pouch, and so on
- Whether the product was meant to be refrigerated, frozen or stored at room temperature

- The lot number, a code revealing the manufacturing plant and production date. (This is a series of letters and numbers stamped on packaging, often near the best by / expiration date, if there is one.)
- The Universal Product Code (UPC)—you know, the bar code
- The product's net weight
- When and where you bought the food in question
- Whether there are any lab results from testing performed on the suspect food
- How the food was stored, prepared and handled
- The suffering species, that is, dog, cat, rabbit, fish, bird, iguana, orangutan, and so on
- The pet's age, weight, breed, whether pregnant, whether spayed or neutered
- Your pet's previous health status
- Any preexisting conditions of your pet
- Whether you give your pet other foods, treats, dietary supplements or drugs
- How much of the suspect food your pet normally consumes
- How much of the product your pet ate just before becoming ill
- How much of the product you still have on hand
- Any outward symptoms such as vomiting, diarrhea, lethargy and the like.
- How soon the symptoms showed up after the meal
- Your vet's contact info, diagnosis and medical records for that pet
- Any results of diagnostic lab testing conducted after your pet got sick
- How many pets exhibited clinical symptoms after eating the product
- Whether any pets remained unaffected by the suspect food
- Whether your pets play outdoors unsupervised
- Reasons why you suspect the food in question actually caused the illness

A Review for You

In this chapter, we really tried stepping back from human fare to get a gander at food-borne perils facing people-dependent pets. But alas, the long and winding road to problematic pet provisions leads inextricably back to food threats to humans.

Think Al Pacino in *The Godfather: Part III*, bemoaning his failure to get the Corleone family out of organized crime: "Just when I thought I was out, they *pull me back in*." What does Michael Corleone have to do with this? The abridged version:

The year 2007 was a watershed for spotlighting the threat posed by pet food. That's when the FDA addressed a growing epidemic of renal (kidney) failure among dogs and cats. The agency traced the problem to wheat-gluten fillers imported from China for use in pet foods. The threat circled back to humans when the government revealed that some of the pet food ended up as feed for livestock ultimately slaughtered for human consumption.

In other words, the threat to an unwitting Fido might also harm humans, although Uncle Sam took pains to soft-pedal any serious compromise of the human food supply.

We also learned that recalls of commercial pet food are as routine as those for human foodstuffs. In looking for an alternative, we looked at the burgeoning raw pet food movement. What we found were passionate advocates both for and against raw diets, which consist of meat, bones, organs, raw eggs and other determinedly natural, uncooked ingredients. Yet both proponents and opponents—the latter including the FDA and respected veterinary medical schools—agree raw diets *pose measurable bacterial threats to pets and their owners.*

"What You Can Do" Checklist: Keeping You and Your Pet Healthy

Buy American

It's not about economic patriotism. Actually, to protect pets as much as possible, make sure your animal food and treats are American-made. Those from

China or elsewhere overseas usually are produced under limited regulations and their safety can't be satisfactorily verified. Your best bet: US-manufactured pet foods, domestically sourced and grown.

Look for organic foods, but avoid those made with flour or anything refined. Best are organics containing only a few healthful, whole foods, such as chicken or brown rice.

And beware of anything containing glycerin, which has been linked to tainted treats.

COMMERCIAL PET FOOD

The FDA advises that to reduce the risk of food-borne illness from commercial pet food, start by buying only those products appearing in good condition in store displays. Reach past the dented cans, torn pouches or discolored bags and go straight for the products in pristine packaging.

PREPARING COMMERCIAL PET FOOD

Remember: "You can't be too clean." Here are some other tips from the FDA:

✓ Wash your hands with soap and hot water for at least twenty seconds before *and after* handling food and treats.
✓ Do the same for pet food bowls and scooping utensils after every use.
✓ Don't use dog or cat bowls to scoop food. Use a clean scoop, spoon or cup. And use it only for scooping pet food. Anything else would be *uncivilized*—not to mention risky.
✓ Dispose of old or spoiled pet food safely by tying it up snugly in a plastic bag and dropkicking the sack into a covered trashcan.

STORING PET FOOD

✓ Got leftover wet pet food—canned or pouched—from Chuckles's recent repast? Either toss or refrigerate it, but move quickly. Know that refrigeration will keep the nastiest bacteria from growing and multiplying and make sure the fridge is at forty degrees Fahrenheit or lower.

A refrigerator thermometer can ease your mind by confirming an accurate interior temp.

✓ Kibble should be stored in a dry place no warmer than eighty degrees Fahrenheit.

✓ The FDA recommends storing dry food in its original bag (with the top folded down), then putting it away inside a clean plastic container with a snap lid.

✓ Keep Fido and Fifi away from wherever you prepare and store their food.

✓ Keep all your four-legged rascals out of trashcans.

RAW PET FOOD

✓ Don't feed your dog or cat raw pet food, either packaged or homemade. The risks are just too high.

Five

How to Keep Dining Out from Becoming a Gross-Out

What are the biggest differences between eating at home and dining out? Well, once you get past décor and ambiance, the big differences probably include the quality, texture, taste, cost and healthfulness of the meal. And about that last one—when it comes to restaurants, one eternal question remains unanswered. And it's one that eats away at just about everyone.

Vengeful Staff: Urban Myth or Everyday Peril?

You've just ordered a meal—after berating, belittling or otherwise verbally bashing your server. Maybe the server had it coming, or maybe you just had a bad day.

Regardless, the moment the waitperson leaves, you're gripped by a figurative fist of fear, the same palpitating panic you've previously

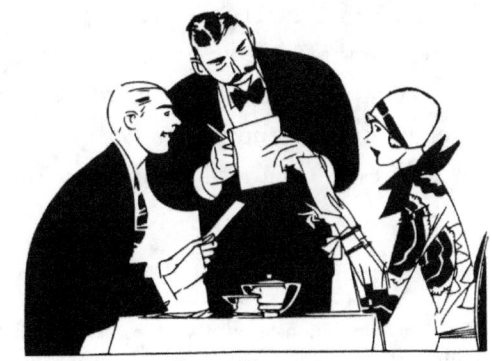

pondered when sending a meal back to the chef: "Will they spit (or worse) on my salmon, just to teach me a lesson?"

Very legit question.

An informal check of the web suggests you're probably safe. For example, in his Yahoo blog *The Sideshow*, Eric Pfeiffer quotes a source inside New York's chichi, pricey French–New American restaurant Per Se: "The cooks work seventy or eighty hours a week and make next to nothing, but they work because they want to cook. And to do that to something, to spit in prep work that someone has spent eight hours of work on—blood, sweat, and tears and all— it's just not done."

On the New York–centric food site BridgeandTunnelClub.com, blogger and veteran waiter Michael Sendrow (a.k.a. Monkey Boy) agrees that sabotaging savories is a rarity: "In all of my years of serving, I have only once seen a retaliation. A particularly feisty coworker at a coffee shop I used to manage got so mad at a regular jerk-ass customer that she once spiked his Americano with Visine®, believing it would give him diarrhea." (Apparently, it does much worse; let's not go there.)

Sendrow says most restaurant workers are just too busy to bother with such tactics. He chalks up public concern to misplaced cynicism. "I can't count the number of times I've heard, 'You're probably going to spit in my food now, huh?' from a difficult customer," Monkey Boy reported. "Get over it, you paranoid freak."

Must've Been Something I Ate...*at the Restaurant*

Do restaurants serve up a hefty percentage of America's food-borne illnesses?

Many people think so, regardless of medical facts that belie the belief. In a federally funded study,[16] nearly a quarter of the 1,500 people surveyed blamed their illnesses on a restaurant meal. And more than half of those restaurant

---

16 Laura R. Green, Carol Selman, Elaine Scallan, Timothy F. Jones, Ruthann Marcus and the EHS-Net Population Survey Working Group, "Beliefs about Meals Eaten Outside the Home as Sources of Gastrointestinal Illness," *Journal of Food Protection* 68, no. 10 (2005): 2184-2189.

finger pointers based their belief on the fact their symptoms began within five hours of eating.

But…many such bugs *don't strike that quickly*. Therefore, the study concluded, people really don't know how long a rotten repast takes to induce illness—so they can't be sure which meals caused their cramps, diarrhea, vomiting or worse.

The study also found that just 8 percent of victims ever reported their illnesses to public health agencies or the suspect restaurants, making it pretty hard to study and perhaps prevent some food-borne outbreaks.

The Fear-Filled Fish Factor

Public perceptions about certain fares can be unfair, but it's clear one cuisine inspires more distrust than most: fish.

SUSHI AND SASHIMI FARE

When sushi and its raw-relative sashimi became hip on American shores a few decades back, many fish lovers fell ill from the bacteria and parasites that can develop quickly in the Japanese delicacies. The FDA stepped in with prepping guidelines and this appeared to do the trick; the number of sushi-related illnesses is now far lower than disorders from contaminated produce such as jalapeño peppers. In fact, among the relatively few cases of sushi poisoning, improperly prepared rice is the culprit more often than the fish itself. For example, rice left at room temperature can produce the *Bacillus cereus* bacterium, which can lead to diarrhea, nausea and vomiting. So hope your hosts get serious about *B. cereus* and prevent it by giving rice an acidic bath in a vinegary solution. This will lower the pH enough to kill those pretty *cereus* microbes.

And keeping the fish safe is as easy as freezing it at either minus-four degrees Fahrenheit for seven days or at minus-thirty-one degrees Fahrenheit for fifteen hours.

Feel the Fugu Fear, Luke

Many diners are content to stick with the more popular, well-known offerings at their local sushi bars. These include the tuna varieties bluefin,[17] big-eye and yellowfin, and other fish such as eel, red snapper (tai), Japanese yellowtail (hamachi) and salmon. But more adventurous diners seek out exotic offerings such as the poisonous puffer fish fugu.

Some master fugu chefs include a little of the poison tetrodotoxin in their finished dishes. We wonder if diners might balk if they knew tetrodotoxin is more than a thousand times deadlier than cyanide! When eaten, it produces a tingly sensation on the lips, which is fine when fugu is properly and safely prepared. If not, the powerful neurotoxin can be fatal.

And a lethal dose is smaller than *the size of a pinhead!* In fact, just one fish could kill thirty otherwise avid fugu fans.

In our chapter-ending checklist, we'll have some simple suggestions for securing safe sushi.

Irradiation: Irresistible or Irridiculous?

A sea change in the fresh-fish debate came in April 2014, when the Food and Drug Administration abruptly changed policy course. The FDA began allowing ionized radiation ("irradiation") treatment on seafood, including raw, frozen, cooked, partially cooked, shelled or dried crustaceans.[18] Also subject to irradiation under the new policy were cooked or ready-to-cook crustaceans processed with spices or small amounts of other food ingredients. Most prominent among the seafood affected are shrimp, crab, lobster, crayfish and prawns.

Legal in many countries, ionizing radiation exposes foods to an energy source that strips electrons from individual atoms. This kills contaminant bacteria and preserves shelf life, among other benefits. Although the name might suggest otherwise, radiation does not turn food radioactive. Only some Cajun

---

17 Bluefin may be on the brink of extinction due to overfishing. In January 2013, the Pew Environmental Group warned that stocks in the western Pacific Ocean—the Bluefin tuna's main spawning ground—had fallen 96 percent.

18 "FDA Allows Ionizing Radiation to Control Food-borne Pathogens in Crustaceans," April 11, 2014, http://www.fda.gov/Food/NewsEvents/ConstituentUpdates/ucm392860.htm.

spices, certain peppers, Dr. No[19] and a gaggle of Mexican hot sauces can do that.

Irradiation kills pathogens including listeria and *E. coli*, plus a powerful bug new to these pages, vibrio. The newcomer, often associated with raw oysters, can make otherwise-healthy people uncomfortable for a while (with diarrhea, etc.). But vibrio can turn lethal for the less than hale, especially those with impaired immune systems or suffering from cancer, diabetes, liver disorders or other serious illnesses.

But irradiation is no panacea; the agency admits the practice "will reduce, but not entirely eliminate, the number of pathogenic (illness causing) micro-organisms in or on crustaceans."[20] The agency urges consumers and restaurants to continue using established food handling, prep and storage practices.

The new rules call for irradiated seafood to be labeled as such—unless it's contained in a processed meal such as a frozen shrimp dinner or a salad. If that's the case, no label is required. Ditto for irradiated seafood at restaurants, so asking if your seafood was zapped probably is a good idea.

Ionizing radiation has been criticized for potentially causing chemical changes in food that differ from natural ones created during cooking with heat. And not everyone was happy about the FDA's new policy. The non-profit advocacy group Food & Water Watch claims zapping more seafood just mitigates the problem of unsanitary seafood processing overseas. Wenonah Hauter, the group's executive director, notes that the United States imports more than 80 percent of its seafood, much of it from Asia and the People's Republic of China. Hauter claims that the Chinese "raise their seafood in squalid conditions" and that irradiation allows "those countries to continue to raise their seafood products in filthy and unsanitary factory fish farms, since irradiation will be used as the 'magic bullet' to make the products safe to

---

19 In the first James Bond film, *Dr. No* (1962), the British secret agent and a female companion, the white-bikini-clad Honey Ryder, are rendered radioactive (and later decontaminated) by the evil title character.

20 "FDA Allows Ionizing Radiation to Control Food-borne Pathogens in Crustaceans," FDA. gov, accessed March 12, 2015, http://www.fda.gov/Food/NewsEvents/ConstituentUpdates/ucm392860.htm.

eat from microbiological contaminants."[21] She also suggested the FDA policy change was politically motivated and tied to international trade talks.

More on seafood risks in chapter 8, when we look at food dangers lurking on your vacation itinerary.

In a Perfect World...

To paraphrase F. Scott Fitzgerald, restaurateurs are different than you and me. (To this, Ernest Hemingway might have responded, "Yes, they make more food."[22]) What's the point? It doesn't matter whether you're at home cooking for one or at Chez Eats cooking for seventy hungry patrons; food safety precautions are pretty universal, applying equally to residential and restaurant kitchens.

But unlike private homes, the law *demands* restaurants stick to fundamental food safety standards. Nobody—from four-star fine-dining establishments to food trucks, supermarket deli counters and that ramshackle falafel stand down the block—is exempt.

Rules Are Rules

Here's a general look at basic rules for food serving operators—set by local, state or federal bureaucracies—aimed at protecting you, your family and your friends:[23]

- Safe sourcing of food or ingredients, that is, ensuring that a retailer's wholesaling purveyors deliver reliably fresh goods
- Safe temperatures for holding both hot and cold foods

---

21 Leah Zerbe, "Are You Eating Irradiated Seafood?" *Rodale News*, April 14, 2014, http://www.rodalenews.com/irradiated-seafood.

22 The widely quoted, yet long-disputed alleged exchange is as follows. Fitzgerald: "The rich are different from you and me." Hemingway: "Yes, they have more money."

23 "Restaurant Safety: What You Should Know," Centers for Disease Control and Prevention, December 16, 2013, http://blogs.cdc.gov/yourhealthyourenvironment/2013/06/12/restaurant-safety-what-you-should-know/.

- Proper cooking temperatures and times, especially for meat, poultry and pork
- Proper handling to prevent cross-contamination
- Proper hand washing by food handlers to prevent contamination, especially of people who may be sick with vomiting or diarrhea

Inspections

Fear is a great motivator. That's especially true for restaurateurs who, by virtue of their chosen trade, live and die by the "I" word. You'd be on edge too if a public health inspector popped in at your house to test whether you're obeying the law. Restaurateurs *have* to worry about surprise inspection visits.

Rules vary between communities, generally on frequency and grading (i.e., "scoring") systems used to rate food service vendors. Some public health agencies use a numerical score; others assign a letter grade and some municipalities merely dumb it down to a pass-fail scale.

Many communities require a full inspection report, with scores publicly posted at eateries. Sometimes restaurants need only post the score or rating, while other times a public health or other regulatory agency will itself post full reports and scores. In some places, the agency will post only the score—and only on the Internet.

You can ask local food safety regulators about the system in your area. A great source of information for tracking down appropriate officials in your area is the Directory of State and Local Officials from the Association of Food and Drug Officials. The directory is on the web at www.dslo.afdo.org.

Having trouble tracking down a café's score or report? Don't be shy—ask the manager for the most recent findings. If there's any noticeable reluctance, that may be all the answer you need.

If not, technology just might hold the answer. In January 2013, Yelp introduced a hundred-point rating system based directly on local government inspection data. The online review site developed the system in conjunction with staff techies from the Cities of San Francisco and New York, with the blessings of the White House. The result is LIVES—Local Inspector

Value-Entry Specification, which translates local health scores for restaurants listed and reviewed by Yelp contributors.

Expanding from the City by the Bay and the Big Apple, Yelp's program is now nationwide, with a standing invitation to all municipalities to participate by sharing restaurant-inspection and hygiene data.

An Ounce of Prevention

So how to stop food poisoning before it starts? Try paraphrasing the mantra employed by driving instructors: Learn to dine defensively.

Pay attention to your surroundings. Develop a healthy skepticism about all the elements of your dine-out experience. And think like a health inspector. Consider these strategies:

- **Visit the great outdoors.** On arrival, look for any visible trash bins out back. Do they teem with trash? Is garbage strewn across the parking lot? A wide-open back door is the restaurant equivalent of a neon sign flashing, "Insects and vermin, enter here." Also, are restaurant workers out back, hosing down floor mats or dumping wastewater on the pavement or nearby? These are practically engraved invitations to roaches and other crawly, carpetbagging visitors. Remember that conditions outside an eatery often reflect the owners' indoor commitment (or lack of it) to cleanliness.

- **Appoint yourself secretary of the interior.** Once inside a restaurant, be wary if floors, walls or decorations appear dusty or dirty; the same goes for tables, chairs, booths and other surfaces. Carpets and rugs should be free of food detritus, grease and stains. Check to see if dishes, silverware, drinking glasses and utensils are free of stains, smudges or lipstick. And look out for cracked or chipped dishware.

- **Don't dance with this salsa.** The zingy south-of-the-border dip may have more kick than the Rockettes. But salsa, along with guacamole, is increasingly causing illness. These favorites often are prepared in large batches and with various ingredients, then improperly refrigerated.

Ever notice what happens to guacamole after it sits out for a few hours? Not a pretty sight—but a solid deterrent to derring-do dipping.

- **Don't order fish on Mondays.** If you do, chances are you'll be eating swimmers at least three days old—which makes the fish *this close* to poisonous. *Food Poison Journal* explains that many restaurants buy fresh fish in anticipation of the big crowds on Saturday nights. By Monday, that same fish is old enough to apply for Social Security retirement benefits.

- **Check out the staff.** Forget the sexy eye contact; repeated exposure to flirty customers has made servers immune to the charms of strangers. Instead, scrutinize waitstaff and chefs for clean aprons and attire, including shoes. If cooks are wiping their hands on their aprons, they're transferring bacteria that can easily find a path straight to your stomach. Also look to see if kitchen chefs and servers are wearing appropriate hairnets and restraints. And are their hands, fingernails and cuticles clean?

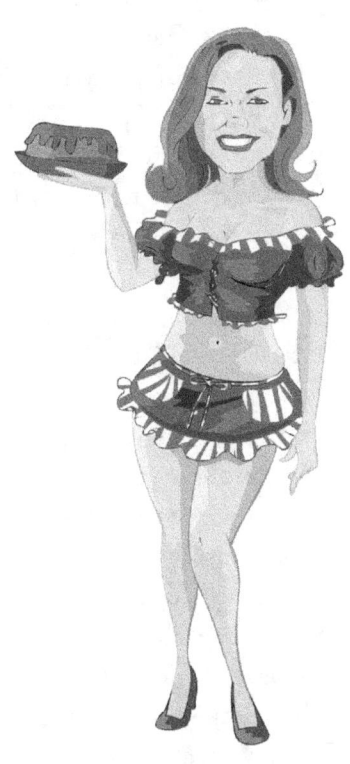

- **Follow your nose.** Be old school—sniff your food. If it doesn't smell or taste right, do you really want to take a risk by not sending it back?

- **Use your eyes, too.** You don't have to be a chef at the Cordon Bleu to recognize when beef, chicken, pork, veal, turkey, pheasant, duck, Cornish game hen, buffalo, elk, mutton, venison or other animal protein is undercooked. If that telltale pink is in the middle, don't put on a brave face. Send it back for more heat.

- **Does dirty bathroom equal yucky kitchen?** A messy bathroom can (though not always) correlate with a filthy kitchen. Restroom conditions can be telling anyway because if the liquid soap (and it definitely should be liquid, not bar soap) isn't refilled, or if the paper towels are gone, remember that this is probably where the staff washes up too.
- **Don't believe there's no such thing as bad publicity.** Other than Queen Elizabeth II, who *doesn't* love hole-in-the-wall joints? But, sad to say, chain restaurants may actually be safer than mom-and-pop spots. Big chain restaurants have the most to lose from bad publicity borne of filthy conditions or toxic food. The financial information website MarketWatch.com reports that, statistically speaking, you're safer eating at a chain outlet because chains have greater resources to devote to food safety and usually impose strict, formal cleanliness standards on employees.

A Review for You

In this chapter, we looked at the myths, perceptions and potential triggers that can motivate vengeful restaurant staffers to use your food as a spittoon.

We also learned that a large segment of the public tends to blame restaurants for their food-borne illnesses, even if their suspicions are undercut by science or common sense. It's no coincidence that the rules governing restaurant procedures are close to those we discussed in earlier chapters about best practices at home, including proper food sourcing, refrigeration, cleanliness and other ways to prevent cross-contamination, spoilage and bacterial dangers.

We peeked at restaurant inspections, the grading of eateries on health and safety practices and how you can find out how your favorite dining spots graded out.

But we saved some of the most meaningful information for last: more practical tips to help make your dining out experience delicious instead of dangerous.

"What You Can Do" Checklist: Dodging Disease at the Deli and Diner

✓ **The bitter truth about lemons.** They're usually dirty because restaurants often don't wash them. Lemons frequently are kept in the shipping box right up until being sliced and served. In fact, slicing an unwashed lemon can contaminate the fruit because anything untoward on the rind—notably bacteria and insecticide residue—gets onto the knife and thus onto the pulp inside. Rind-ridin' germs can include mold, bacteria, staph and Candida yeast, the last one found in the mouth and, gulp, certain places on the female body. Solution: Always order lemons on the side. Squeeze them into your drink or onto that slab o' salmon—but don't let the juice come in contact with the rind.

✓ **Beware the buffet.** Sure, cafeteria-style dining is a way of life at resorts and vacation destinations like Vegas. But buffets are also factories for bad germs—*facteria for bacteria*. Since many hot foods cool their heels for hours in chafing dishes of inconsistent temperatures, the stuff on the bottom often burns, while topside food can get cold. Also, buffets sometimes use artificial ingredients like fake eggs. Solution: If you can't resist the lure of all-you-can-eat,[24] minimize the risk and dine when the buffet first opens; you'll get the highest level of freshness. For lunch, try arriving at noon; at dinnertime, aim for 5:00 p.m.

✓ **All-you-can-avoid.** In theory, an all-you-can-eat buffet seems like a gastronomic paradise. But beware: It often means you're satisfying yourself silly with low-quality foods—cheaper cuts of meat or items stuffed with starch or filled with fat.

✓ **The "daily special": an oxymoron?** Too often, the special is anything but. Sometimes, it's a culinary dumping ground of aging meat and fish, old vegetables and yesterday's sauces—all the leftovers a chef wants to use up before they break completely bad. Solution: If the daily special sounds good to you, quiz your server about the ingredients.

---

24 Or, as we often described Aunt Esther's dreaded Sunday dinners, all you can *stand.*

Be thorough but polite, lest you become seized by that figurative fist of fear described at the top of the chapter.

✓ **When is veal not real?** Strictly speaking, there's no direct health threat here. We just wanted you to know that restaurants sometimes play fast and loose with their food facts by swapping out the poor man's protein, pork, for the more expensive veal. Once pounded, dressed in breadcrumbs or swimming in sauce, pork can pass for veal, at least among less discerning palettes. (Indeed, some places play similar bait and switch involving Kobe beef, sushi and various high-end seafood.)

✓ **A word about veal.** Just don't do it. Don't order veal in restaurants or cook it at home. Just forget about it. In a veal-less world, there would be no veal industry to raise nearly a million otherwise unwanted calves, animals cruelly chained up in severely confined wooden crates so small they can't even turn around. Veal calves are fed a nutrient-deficient liquid diet that leaves their muscles underdeveloped—solely to produce a pale-colored meat at slaughter time. Veal calves are slaughtered between just sixteen and twenty weeks of age.[25] We could go on and on, but you get the idea. If you care at all about animals, please resist just one animal protein in this life: veal.

✓ **Dinner *before* eight.** Fred Astaire movies and New York socialites make late dining seem glamorous. But it might also be dangerous. The closer it gets to closing time, the likelier your meal will be bacterially suspect. After all, the ingredients were prepared hours earlier, giving germs plenty of time to mess with your meal. And the kitchen may be in a similarly scary state. For example, the fryers are full of sludge that began the day as fresh cooking oil, and the kitchen staff likely has shifted into cleanup mode, so an errant cleaning spray could mist your meat or season your soufflé. Solution: If dining late, order something grilled, broiled or boiled. At least your food won't be raw and therefore more vulnerable to bacterial invaders.

---

25 All information presented here concerning the raising and treatment of calves bred for veal producers is from the Massachusetts Society for the Prevention of Cruelty to Animals via the website MSPCA.org.

✓ **Pack yourself up, dust yourself off, eat all over again.** Got leftovers? Don't leave it to your server or a passing busboy to box up your dinner's delicious detritus. If your food is transferred in the kitchen, it'll probably share counter space with dirty dishes or be within spitting distance of garbage. And if your dinner roll fell to the floor before being stashed in your leftovers container, would you even know it? Solution: Insist on packing up the leftovers yourself. And remember: Using a doggie bag is a crapshoot. High-risk food left in the temperature danger zone—41 to 140 degrees Fahrenheit—is at serious risk of bacterial contamination. Ditto if the consumer either handles leftovers improperly or reheats them inadequately.

✓ **What's on the menu tonight?** Well, just about everything from fecal bacteria like *E. coli* to *Streptococcus* and more. That's because menus themselves aren't properly wiped down often enough and are touched by countless hands in an average day. Solution: Handle the menu by the top corners instead of at the bottom like most people do. You'll evade exposure to a big chunk of the little devils.

✓ **Fountains of sorrow.** If carbonated sodas aren't healthful—and seriously, they're not—the fountains dispensing them at fast food outlets, convenience stores and elsewhere are downright nasty. According to a 2010 study published in the *International Journal of Food Microbiology*,[26] 48 percent of sodas tested from thirty fountains in Virginia contained coliform bacteria. That family of teeny, humorless miscreants (including *E. coli*) is found in the feces of warm-blooded animals. Yep—even more fecal matter to ponder. Worse, at least seven other pathogens also turned up, most of them antibiotic resistant. Solution: Illnesses traced directly to soda fountains are rare. But to be safe, if you can choose between a fountain drink and a beverage in a bottle or can—go with the latter.

---

26 Amy S. White, Renee D. Godard, Carolyn Belling, Victoria Kasza and Rebecca L. Beach, "Beverages Obtained from Soda Fountain Machines in the U.S. Contain Microorganisms, Including Coliform Bacteria," *International Journal of Food Microbiology* 137, no. 1 (2010): 61-66.

✓ **Suggestions for safe sushi.** Trust the pros. Your safest sushi bets are found at restaurants or in sushi containers from the supermarket. If you insist on preparing your own sushi, buy the frozen, sushi-grade fish—the quality stuff, not cheaper, inferior cuts—per FDA regulations. Eat your sushi as soon as you can and don't let leftovers hang around in the fridge for more than twenty-four hours.

Six

No "Maybe Baby" When You're Talking Food Safety

Most mothers probably would agree that when it comes to baby safety, you can't be too fearful, obsessive or paranoid. Comes with the territory, right? While the following tale isn't food related, it's a classic example:

We know a couple whose newborn daughter never slept through the night, waking every few hours. One night, to her mother's horror, two-month-old Louise fell asleep around eleven—and didn't wake up! This was unheard-of for an infant frequently driven around for hours in the dead of night just so the car's gentle rocking would lull her to sleep.

By eight the following morning, Louise's panicked parents left a frantic message with their pediatrician's exchange. Then, they waited and paced, paced and waited.

A few minutes later, the doctor called back with a simple question: "Have you tried waking her up?"

"Yes, yes, yes...*of course!*" (Translation: "You can't possibly think we're that stupid, can you?")

"Try again."

They did. Sure enough, little Louise opened her eyes, offered an innocent yawn and smiled sweetly at her gobsmacked parents.

"Fortunately," Louise's mother, cringing once again, recalled a dozen years later, "when we told the doctor a moment later, we *didn't* hear laughter coming back from the other end of the line."

Moral of the story: sometimes you can't be too careful, even when risking

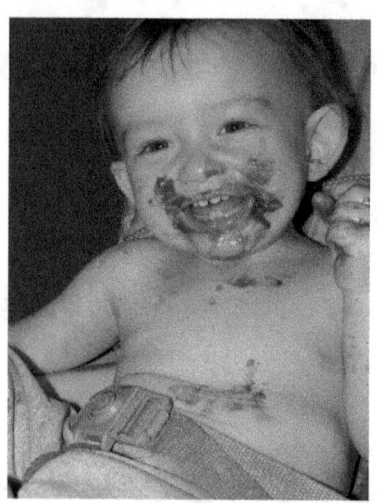

appearing foolish. And while this chapter is all about food, not sleep, the Louise rule is especially appropriate here. If any of our advice seems overcautious, we plead guilty.

This chapter is meant as a quick-reference feeding guide for new and recent parents because infants and younger children are especially susceptible to food-borne illness—their young immune systems haven't sufficiently developed to guard against infections. Naturally, your pediatrician or a pediatric nutritionist can offer far more detailed information and advice.

Milk? Just Say No

Got milk? If it's for baby, forget it. According to the multiagency federal website FoodSafety.gov, cow's milk is bad news for babies under a year old. It lacks the proper nutritional balance for infants to grow normally; worse, it can promote anemia and hinder kidney function.

And raw (a.k.a. "fresh" or "fresh unprocessed," i.e., unpasteurized[27]) milk is even less trustworthy—and not just for the little ones. FoodSafety.gov warns that nobody should drink, sip, slurp, gulp, lap up, ingest or otherwise swallow raw milk. Ever. Unless they like exposing themselves to salmonella, *E. coli* and listeria.

---

27   In pasteurization, milk is heated either to 145 degrees Fahrenheit for a half hour or 163 degrees Fahrenheit for fifteen seconds. The process kills certain (although not all) bacteria and effectively deactivates some enzymes, with minimal harm to the taste.

According to muckraking magazine *Mother Jones,*[28] raw milk's ardent advocates insist it contains life-affirming enzymes and probiotics.[29] And it's no big shock that raw's most vocal boosters include Organic Pastures of Fresno, California, the nation's largest raw milk producer. *Mother Jones* quoted the company's CEO, Mark McAfee, on raw's alleged restorative powers: "People see amazing results when they give this stuff to their kids—they have ear infections and asthma and allergies, and with raw milk it goes away."

Verifiable proof of this, however, remains elusive.

What isn't questionable is the high-profile case of Chris Martin of Murrieta, California. In 2006, the then seven-year-old picked up *E. coli* from tainted raw milk. He nearly died. After his kidneys failed, Chris spent two months in the hospital—and faced the potential of serious side effects for many years.

So our take on raw milk: The cow says, *mooooo*; we just say, *nooooo*.

Breast Milk

Health experts generally agree breast milk is better for baby than formula. In fact, both the World Health Organization (WHO) and the American Academy of Pediatrics (AAP) urge that infants be exclusively breast-fed for the first six months of life. WHO describes this as "the best start for [babies'] growth, development and health."

Both the AAP and the respected global nonprofit La Leche League say that at room temperature—sixty-six to seventy-two degrees Fahrenheit—breast milk will keep safely for six to eight hours. The groups also agree refrigerated breast milk should stay fresh for two to three days, although La Leche actually goes much further, declaring it should remain safe in the fridge for up to eight days.

Freezing breast milk is perfectly fine. The American Academy of Breastfeeding Medicine reports frozen mother's milk can remain fresh and

---

28 Kiera Butler, "Is Raw Milk Really Good for You?" *Mother Jones*, Sept./Oct. 2012, accessed March 10, 2015, http://www.motherjones.com/environment/2012/09/is-raw-milk-safe-e-coli.

29 The so-called "good bacteria." More detail on probiotics in chapter 10.

healthful for three to six months—if frozen at zero degrees Fahrenheit in a refrigerator freezer with its own separate door. The milk should be stored near the back of the freezer, where temperature is most constant. It can be safely frozen for longer periods, but some lipids in the milk will degrade, undercutting the milk's quality.[30]

Formula

Most brands of infant formula—the chief stand-in for breast milk—are derived from cow's milk. Not to worry—the milk in formula is modified with supplemental nutrients to ensure it's healthful and more easily digested than pure cow's milk.

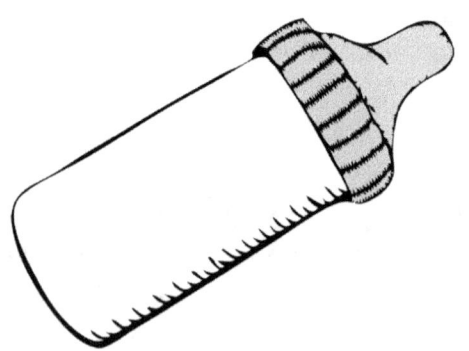

There's also soy-based formula, which the AAP says accounts for about a fifth of all infant formula sold in the United States. Some parents and physicians insist soy helps with colic, diarrhea, allergies and eczema. But the AAP disputes most of these claims, recommending soy-based formula for only a select few: infants who are lactose intolerant, from strict vegan families or suffering from the rare condition galactosemia, which makes the body unable to metabolize the naturally occurring sugar galactose.

Other formula varieties include a hypoallergenic mixture and formula for preterm ("preemie") babies or those with other health issues. Formula is available powdered and in liquid varieties, including ready to feed and liquid concentrates.

---

30 Academy of Breastfeeding Medicine Protocol committee, "Human Milk Storage Information for Home Use for Full-Term Infants," *Breastfeed Medicine* 5, no. 3 (2010): 127-30.

Equipment Care and Handling

No surprises here: Before handling feeding equipment, wash your hands thoroughly with soap and hot water and use a clean cloth to dry them. Then wash all equipment completely in hot soapy water.

Use a bottle and teat brush to really scrub the feeding bottles, teats and lids, inside and out; you don't want leftover bits of food hiding in nooks and crannies. Then, sterilize everything by submerging all the newly scrubbed components in a big covered pot of water, making sure no air bubbles get trapped. Bring to a hearty boil, then keep everything in the covered pan until baby is hungry and the equipment is needed.

Of course, don't forget to turn off the burner after the boil begins, and don't touch newly sterilized equipment without scrubbing your hands again. The WHO also recommends sterilized forceps to handle the newly germless equipment.

If you take the items from the sterilizing pot before needing them, fully assemble the bottles to prevent new contamination and keep them covered and out of the way.

No Nukes!

Don't be tempted to use a microwave oven as a shortcut to prep or reheat breast milk or formula. Microwaves may be great for popcorn or frozen burritos, but they heat unevenly and may create "hot spots" that could scald your child's mouth.

Baby's Own Twelve-Step Program

It's not what you think—unless you regard bottled formula as baby's own drinking problem. Here's how the WHO recommends prepping a bottle-feed:

1. **Clean and disinfect** the surface (countertop, e.g.) on which you'll be working.
2. **Wash those hands** thoroughly, just like we told you before. If you skip this important step, you risk exposing baby to bad bugs you may

have picked up from touching raw meat, poultry, seafood, eggs, dirty diapers, family pets and who knows what else.

3. **Prep safe water.** Heat tap or bottled water to a roiling boil;[31] then let it bubble for another minute; you can forgo this step only if the bottled water's label indicates it's sterile. In general, bottled water is neither sterile nor safer (before boiling) than regular tap water. After boiling, let the water cool to body temperature before mixing. The World Health Organization maintains water must be down to at least seventy degrees Fahrenheit before being mixed with powdered formula to kill the dangerous *Cronobacter* bacterial genus.

4. **With formula, check packaging** for the correct amounts of water and powder to mix. Don't try to adjust the ratio for larger or smaller amounts. This might seem intuitive, but messing with measurements could make your baby ill.

5. **Pour the correct volume** of boiled (sterilized) water into the lovingly cleaned and sterilized feeding bottle.

6. **Add the precise amount** of formula to the bottle.

7. **Gently shake** or swirl the bottle.

8. **Cool the mixture to feeding temperature** by either holding the bottle under cold running water or in a container of cold or iced water. But don't risk contamination—keep the cooling water below the bottle's lid.

9. **Dry the bottle's exterior** with a clean or disposable cloth.

10. **Drip a little feed** onto the inside of your wrist. You're looking for lukewarm; if it's still hot, cool it down some more before feeding.

11. **Let baby have it.**

12. **Any leftover liquid?** Toss it within two hours.

The Finer Points of Formula

- **Be careful.** Formula is stunningly susceptible to bacterial contamination during preparation. In fact, the WHO reports that because

---

31 Don't confuse this with an angry monarch, or "boiling royal."

powdered infant formula is not a sterile product, it can contain the potentially lethal group of bacteria mentioned above called *Cronobacter* (for many years known as *Enterobacter sakazakii*). The illness it causes is rare—the CDC gets wind of just a few infant cases a year—but very scary, capable of causing sepsis (severe blood infections), meningitis (an inflammation of membranes protecting the spine and brain) or both. Those facing the greatest risk include infants less than two months of age—especially preemies—plus low-birth-weight babies and babies with compromised immune systems.

- **To mix safely, make smaller quantities as needed.** This will slash the chance of bacterial squatters moving in and multiplying exponentially. And always faithfully follow product instructions for mixing. If you don't use the formula right away, refrigerate it immediately. Place any leftover liquid in the fridge posthaste; dallying on this risks bacterial contamination.
- **Says WHO.** The World Health Organization recommends "full traceability" of prepared formula by labeling every container of mixed formula with its type, the baby's name or ID, the preparer's name and the date and time it was prepared. Again, you can't be too careful.
- **For high-risk infants, go liquid.** Use sterile liquid infant formula if available.

Juice Box (and Pouch) Sanity

Early in its long TV run, the opening of *Everybody Loves Raymond* immortalized a struggle most real-life parents encounter. Costar Patricia Heaton, as wife and mom Debra Barone, fails to spike a kid's single-serve juice box with its accompanying mini straw. She just can't seem to puncture the box's small, foil-covered hole.

We feel her pain. But beyond uncooperative straw holes, these juice boxes can pose a danger, especially to the biggest market for these drinks—kids.

Nobody wants to discover, midsip, that they're drinking moldy juice from an innocent-looking container. So before you sip, find the expiration date. If you are way past it, why risk illness? Chuck the container into the next county.

Next, check the outside of the box or pouch for signs of dried juice, stains, moisture or anything else suggesting leakage or problematic packaging. To paraphrase a famous criminal attorney, if you have any doubt, toss it out.[32]

Still on the freshness fence? Snip open the top and look inside for signs of mold or anything else compromising the juice. If your fears are confirmed, toss the container right away. Don't even sniff the contents—mold spores can cause respiratory problems. Sure, snipping cancels the convenience of single-serving packages. But if the contents are still fresh, you can down the drink via straw or by going old school: tilt the package and gulp away.

And you won't even have to struggle with stabbing the little hole.

One Hundred Years of Solid Food[33]

Actually, it's nearly two full centuries since Europe's industrial revolution introduced mass production of baby foods, starting with infant formulae developed by scientists and nutrition experts of that time. By the 1920s, according to FoodTimeline.org, the list of mass-produced baby foods had expanded to include cereals, fruits and vegetables.

During those halcyon days of hootch, flappers and Clara Bow, the Madison Avenue marketing men already were pushing the selling point of convenience. They also preyed on the public's rationalistic side—people's faith in science—by steering mothers away from the homemade stuff and toward "modern, scientifically formulated" manufactured baby foods.

These days, we know much more about healthful infant and toddler diets than we did in the Roaring Twenties. Back then, both malted milk and chocolate pudding were marketed as *health foods* for kids.

---

32 At O. J. Simpson's criminal trial in 1996, a notorious pair of bloody gloves led lead defense attorney Johnnie Cochran to coin the now-famous phrase, "If it doesn't fit, you must acquit."
33 Apologies to Gabriel García Márquez, Nobel Prize–winning author of *One Hundred Years of Solitude*.

We'll have safety tips on solid baby foods in our checklist at chapter's end.

Meantime, empowered with modern nutritional information, many parents today are returning to an earlier baby food tradition.

DIY for the Small Fry

Before mass production, baby food usually was made at home. These days, homemade is enjoying a renaissance as plenty of parents whip up fresh, nutritious baby foods inexpensively in home kitchens. Those ubiquitous guys in baby food marketing can only look on forlornly.

The FDA's Office of Food Safety suggests these steps for selecting, preparing and storing homemade baby food.

Selecting ingredients. Use fresh items whenever you can, although frozen or canned items will do as backups. If you must use processed fruits or veggies, look for products without added sugar. That's especially true for canned fruit, often packed in sweetened syrup so thick it makes motor oil look runny.

Never use the following, either in homemade baby food or by themselves:

- Any dairy products made from raw, unpasteurized milk
- Honey, which puts babies under a year old at high risk for botulism, the potentially fatal paralytic illness
- Food from dented, rusted, bulging or leaking cans or jars, which, if infiltrated by simple air, can also harbor the bacterium causing botulism (especially vulnerable are cans of low-acid veggies, including green beans, corn, beets and peas)
- Home-canned food, which if not properly sealed can contain dangerous bacteria
- Outdated canned food
- Any food from cans or jars without labels

Preparing the baby food. A zillion websites provide easy and nutritious recipes. We don't endorse any particular site, but know that a simple online search will produce many options and ideas. In general, here are some rules when doing it yourself:

- Wash those hands. Thoroughly. We won't tell you again.
- Use separate cutting boards for meat, poultry and fish and for non-meat foods to prevent cross contamination.
- Wash fresh fruits and vegetables under running water. Plan to peel something? Wash the outside anyway. As we've said, slicing an unwashed item can transfer bacteria from the knife to the fruit inside.
- Again, follow the rules for slapping silly those dastardly bacteria inside popular proteins: meats must be cooked to an internal temperature of at least 160 degrees Fahrenheit, fish to at least 145 degrees Fahrenheit and white-meat poultry to a minimum of 165 degrees Fahrenheit. Don't forget the meat thermometer you'll need to confirm these temps.

A Review for You

In this chapter's look at baby food safety, we underscored that cow's milk not only lacks critical nutritional components but also can lead to anemia and kidney problems. And we don't recommend raw—that is, unpasteurized—milk, either, due to the risk of bacterial contamination.

When it comes to fulfilling nutritional needs, breast milk remains baby's go-to food. For infants, it's everything cow's milk isn't—namely, balanced and nutritionally rich.

Man-made liquid formula is an acceptable alternative because while formula does contain cow's milk, it has undergone considerable nutritional fortification.

Prepping bottles is all about clean and sterile. First, scrub your hands in hot, soapy water. Then do the same with the bottle components. Boil everything—except your hands—into the *good kind of sterility*. Later on, don't touch newly sterilized equipment without repeating the hand-scrubbing routine.

We nixed nuking baby food—formula or solid—in the microwave because unlike cell phone hot spots, the food hot spots produced by these ovens can burn baby's tender mouth in mere moments.

We also provided a simple, twelve-step instruction for bottle feeding, some general info about solid food and some basic advice on making it safely at home.

"What You Can Do" Checklist: Baby Food Basics

FORMULA LIFESPANS

- ✓ **Pristine, never-opened containers** of powdered, ready-to-feed and concentrated liquid formula should be used by the "sell by" or "use by" date. Yes, in chapter 2 we told you neither of those dates was carved in stone. But when it comes to your baby's development, it's better to err on the side of caution.
- ✓ **Opened cans of powdered formula** will keep for a month when the lid is screwed on tightly, unless otherwise specified by the manufacturer, according to the American Academy of Pediatrics. Note: You probably don't want to store it in the fridge, lest you risk a case of clumping.
- ✓ **Opened cans of ready-to-feed and liquid-concentrate** formula are usable up to forty-eight hours if kept tightly covered in the fridge.
- ✓ **Prepared bottles of powdered formula** will keep safely up to twenty-four hours if refrigerated.
- ✓ **Unrefrigerated bottles** should be used within two hours. If you need to keep them out of the refrigerator for more than two hours, keep them chilled with a cold pack in an insulated bag.
- ✓ **Leftover formula in a bottle** shouldn't be saved in the bottle for later—bacterial growth can develop quickly from baby's mouth germs. Transfer right away to a fresh bottle.

✓ **A day's supply of bottles** can safely be prepped all at once. Keep them in the fridge until needed; place them at the back to minimize warm-air exposure when opening the refrigerator door.

SHHH! SECRETS OF THE FORMULA TRADE

✓ **Rinse off and towel dry a powdered container's top** before first opening it to prevent dust or dirt on the lid from getting inside.

✓ **Expressly follow** the manufacturer's mixing instructions for powder-to-water ratio.

✓ *Never* **freeze formula.** This means *you.*

✓ **Skip the sniff.** Don't rely on your finely honed sense of smell to decide whether formula is safe—contamination can be odorless, silent and *insidiously sneaky.*

SOLID-FOOD LIFESPANS

Most unopened jars of solid baby food can be kept at room temperature in a cupboard, no prob—or on a countertop, in the broom closet, hidden in grandma's antique Bavarian cookie jar or in any similarly benign place.

Some brands of organic or flash-frozen baby foods are sold from store freezers or fridges for a reason: they must always be chilled. So once you get them home, they still require cold storage, including any untouched leftovers from baby's elegant repast.

For opened jars, shelf life varies depending on the type of baby food involved (but note that freezing opened food always requires a separate freezer compartment with its own door):

✓ **Strained fruits and vegetables** keep just fine in the fridge for up to three days; in the freezer, they're good for six to eight months.

✓ **Strained meats** can be trusted for just a day in the fridge; in the freezer, they're good for a month or two.

✓ **Meat/veggie combos** get one or two good days in the refrigerator, and in the freezer, a month, maybe two.

More Solid Advice

- ✓ **No nukes, redux.** Don't microwave baby food jars. Just don't do it. If you must heat a jar's contents, spoon them into a microwave-safe dish or container, heat and stir well. Then test a bit on your wrist for temperature. But use a fresh spoon when segueing from feeling to feeding.
- ✓ **Don't spoon serve straight from the jar,** not if there's leftover food you'll use later; baby's saliva can easily contaminate the jar's contents. First, spoon food into a separate dish just before serving; then save what's left in the jar.
- ✓ **With solid, homemade baby food,** freeze it into cubes in an ice-cube tray, then pop the little suckers out and store 'em in freezer-safe plastic bags.
- ✓ **From our bulging "you can't be too safe or too paranoid" file,** inspect the inside rims of newly opened jars for cracks or chips—they could indicate the presence of glass shards. Toss away any suspect jars. Likewise, don't buy jars that are sticky. And make darn sure the safety button on a jar's lid is *down.* If the lid doesn't pop up cheerfully on opening, toss the treacherous jar.

Storing and Reheating

- ✓ **Never leave cooked baby food** sitting around at room temperature for more than a couple hours—or a single hour if the weather is over ninety degrees Fahrenheit.
- ✓ **Reheat food** from the fridge or freezer to an internal temp of 165 degrees Fahrenheit.
- ✓ **Don't dare defrost** frozen baby food in standing water or leave it at room temperature.
- ✓ **Psst! Hey! Yeah, you. You wanna date?** Of course you do—if it involves freezing baby food. Label and date your containers of fresh baby food. You can successfully freeze the stuff for up to a month.

The Last Word

We want to stress that the proper care and feeding of newborns, infants and toddlers is far more elaborate than can be covered in a few pages. We urge expectant or new mothers to use this chapter as an overview; for greater detail and instructions, please consult a pediatrician or pediatric nutritionist.

Seven

SURVIVING FOOD TRUCKS, FARMERS' MARKETS, FAIRS, HOLIDAYS AND VACATIONS

So far, we've covered food safety for adults and infants, both at home and when dining out. But life's culinary adventures pop up in so many other venues, bringing with them any number of food (and fun) poisoning agents. You've got to be prepared for dicey dining wherever you find it. Here are some common places where dangers lurk.

Food Trucks (née "Roach Coaches")

Time and familiarity have a way of sanding down the rough edges of popular perception. Movies are good at pointing this out. Like in *Casablanca*, when Humphrey Bogart muses cynically about two murdered couriers: "Yesterday, they were just two German clerks. Today they're the '*honored dead.*'"

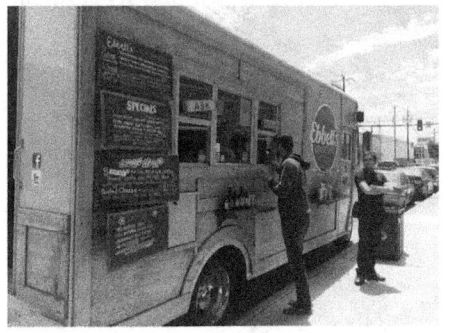

We mention this just to spotlight the latter-day respectability of what used to be called "roach coaches."

These, of course, are food trucks—those ubiquitous, self-contained rolling kitchens once reserved primarily for blue-collar job sites. Nowadays, these tricked-out takeout trucks draw curbside crowds at office parks, high rises, museums and other white-collar haunts, where they serve up a vast variety of fancy-britches fare—from crepes and Mediterranean savories to hipped-up gourmet spins on traditional roach-coach standbys like tacos, pizza and burgers.

But the twenty-first-century mobile-kitchen experience doesn't assure there's been a matching upgrade on food safety. So here are a few pointers to protect yourself from the potential perils of creative mobile pantries and their goose-pâté tacos, cinnamon- and cayenne-accented nouvelle gnocchi and salted-caramel corned-beef kabobs drizzled with raspberry sauce.

- **Local health laws.** Mobile food trucks are regulated by government rules set by your city, county, district or state. You can verify individual truck food licenses, existing local laws and guidelines by contacting your local health department.
- **Food temperatures.** Food should be served at the right thermometer reading; the wrong hot or cold temp can tempt germs to multiply maniacally. Be wary of any hot food you ordered that isn't sufficiently hot when it reaches your hands.
- **Not so touchy!** Truck employees handling food should avoid directly touching your imminent lunch with bare hands. To do so is to risk contaminating not only the food, but also those who consume it *and* anyone in close contact with the soon to be sick. In most jurisdictions, food handlers are required to wear ultrathin, synthetic disposable gloves or to use tongs, other utensils, wax paper and various protective kitchen materials.
- **It's all about you.** We just want to remind *you*, too, to wash your hands before eating or drinking. Unclean hands can cause you to infect your own meal, no matter how careful food-truck chefs might be.

Farmers' Markets

Why have weekly outdoor community markets seen such an explosion of popularity? Could it have something to do with the fresh, crisp vegetables and sweet, juicy fruit delivered straight from the fields? Or the chance to sample a zillion cuisines, many sizzling on portable grills? Maybe it's the world of hot and cold side dishes, homemade juices, candies, legumes, specialties, pies— you name it. And with no middleman, everything sells (theoretically) at near-wholesale prices.

If a farmers' market isn't the closest thing to heaven, what is? As of August 2013, there were a whopping 8,144 farmers' markets regularly staged in the United States, an increase of nearly *fivefold* since 1994. But

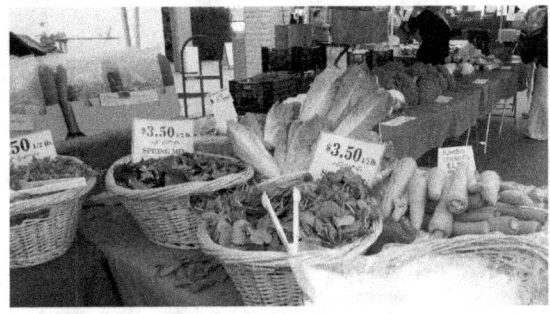

freshness aside, these outdoor food bazaars can pose risks if you're not careful. Here's how the FDA suggests minimizing potential dangers.

- **Meat.** Cuts of meat should be kept in closed coolers with sufficient ice to maintain the low-tech but critical chill factor. Bring an insulated bag (or cooler) with you to keep your purchase cold for the trip home. And keep meat separate from other edibles so the raw juices and their disease-spreadin' bacteria don't mess with the produce and other foods you bought.
- **Eggs.** Don't buy them if they're not kept refrigerated at the market. The FDA mandates untreated shell eggs be stored and displayed at forty-five degrees Fahrenheit. And unless a carton is shrink-wrapped, don't skip the traditional inspection routine of peeking inside to confirm the eggs are clean and the shells unbroken.
- **Milk and cheeses.** After all our warnings about raw milk and salmonella, *E. coli* and listeria, it's no wonder we discourage the purchase of dairy products at farmers' markets—unless you can verify the milk and other products have been pasteurized. And among unpasteurized soft cheeses, feta, Brie, Camembert, blue-veined varieties, queso blanco, queso fresco and queso panela are especially prone to carrying listeria.

- **Produce.** Before and after touching fresh produce, scrub your hands with soap and warm water for twenty seconds. Wash fruits and vegetables under running water before you chop, cook or eat them. And the FDA discourages using soap, detergent or commercial produce washes; a good watery rubdown should do it. But beware of the pineapple's spiky exterior—it's an owie waiting to happen. As we've pointed out before, if you're a-peelin' or a-slicin', always wash an item first—to prevent any bacteria on the outside from transferring to the pulp inside, either from your hand or from the knife you're using. And always refrigerate any cut-up fruit or veggies within two hours.
- **Juices and cider.** Remember what we've said about pasteurized dairy products? Same goes here. If a fruit- or vegetable-based beverage hasn't been pasteurized, confirm it's either in a pressurized container or is cold-pressed. Still, the best practice remains the bacteria-squishing heating process pioneered by nineteenth-century microbiologist Louis Pasteur.[34]

And just because a juice is fresh squeezed doesn't necessarily guarantee safety. When squeezed, a fruit or vegetable's dangerous bacteria can end up in the resulting juice or cider. Be careful to verify that at some point, somebody cleaned up these innocent-looking edibles. If you're unsure about a particular juice or cider, check the label (if there is one) or simply ask. No one will look askance at you; vigilance in the avoidance of bacteria is no vice.

Fairs and Festivals

Food-borne illnesses soar in summer in part because of fairs, festivals, picnics, rodeos and other outdoor, weather-friendly moveable feasts. Mobile food trucks play a part, along with barbecues and other makeshift kitchens lacking routine indoor controls such as thermostat-controlled cooking, refrigeration and the cleaning and sterilizing facilities required of conventional, stationary restaurants.

---

34 Portrayed in the 1936 Warner Bros. biopic by Paul Muni, winner of the Academy Award® as best actor for his performance.

Bringing your own food to the fair? Apply the usual safety standards for handling and storage times. Food shouldn't sit out for more than two hours. If it's hot outside—ninety degrees Fahrenheit or above—cut that to an hour. And keep perishables in a cooler or insulated bag.

Plan to sample the delicious-looking fair fare? Keep reading.

VENDOR? I BARELY *KNOW* 'ER!

You're staring at a trio of vixenish vendors, all seductively beckoning you like the sexy sirens of ancient Greece to try their mind-bending specialties. What should you look for while choosing between the bodacious beef burrito, the chunky-chewy chowder and the sensationally savory salmon? Consider:

- Is the vendor's workstation clean and tidy?
- Is there a sink for food handlers and other employees to wash their hands?
- Do the food handlers wear gloves or use tongs?
- Is there on-site refrigeration for raw ingredients or precooked foods?
- Is there proof the vendor has passed a recent inspection by local health officials?
- Is the vendor's license to sell food and beverages up to date? Laws do differ between states, but temporary and mobile food vendors at fairs and festivals usually are required to obtain food licenses from state or county health departments. Community-based charitable organizations selling edibles at festivals and fairs should also strongly consider obtaining a license.

PETTING ZOOS AND OTHER TOUCHING EXPERIENCES

Kids love makeshift animal habitats at fairs and festivals because they can commune with goats, sheep, ponies and other pettable pals. There's a fine line, however, between communing and contamination. Humans can pick up *more than seventy-five diseases* from contact with animals. In fact, in 2000,

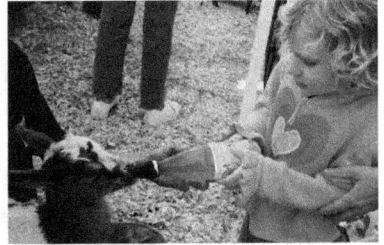

the Centers for Disease Control traced fifty-five cases of *E. coli*, most involving children, to a Pennsylvania petting zoo. Sixteen victims were hospitalized and one, a four-year-old girl, ended up needing a kidney transplant from her father.[35]

The CDC suggests these tips to keep you and the family from becoming statistics:

- Scout out hand-washing stations at fairs, festivals, rodeos and the like.
- Bring hand sanitizers or disposable wipes with you, just in case you can't find a place to wash your hands.
- Wash hands immediately after petting animals, touching their enclosures or leaving animal areas—even if you never actually touch the critters.
- Remember to use soap and clean water for at least twenty seconds.
- Wash those same hands after visiting the restroom, playing a game, going on a ride, eating or drinking, fixing food or drinks, changing a diaper or removing dirty clothes.

Healthy Holidays

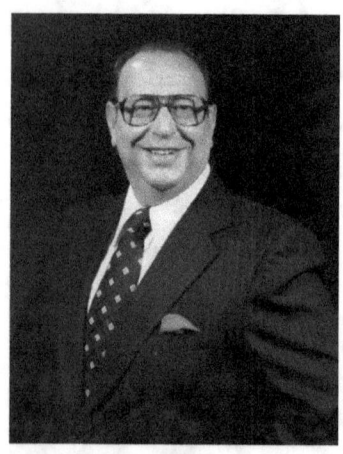

Uncle Phil: a man
and his frosting.

Ah, what's better for the human spirit and for celebrating shared blessings than gathering beloved family and cherished friends at Thanksgiving to eat hearty…and renew lifelong arguments, nurse ancient grudges and engage in petty, personal backbiting and vicious food fights?

Well, family relations aside, at least we can help with food safety around the belt-loosening days of November and December. And make no mistake—the holidays render people especially vulnerable to food-borne illness. Remember, winter is cold and flu season. So between sneezy Mom cooking up a storm and

35 The Humane Society of the United States, "Health Dangers at Petting Zoos and Fairs," Dec. 17, 2009, http://www.humanesociety.org/issues/zoos/facts/health_dangers_petting_zoos.html.

feverish Uncle Phil sneaking a fingerful of frosting, the holiday dinner can morph into a breeding ground of pain.

Remember also that Thanksgiving, Christmas, Hanukkah, Kwanzaa and Festivus usually involve more dishes to heat or chill than the oven or refrigerator can accommodate. This means the cook must develop military-caliber precision to keep everything properly heated or chilled so bacteria doesn't settle into stuffing, tour the turkey, groove with the gravy and primp inside the pumpkin pie.

Complicating the seasonal issue is that holiday gatherings are packed with the people most vulnerable to food-borne illness and whose immune systems are most easily compromised—the elderly, young people and pregnant women. So the need for care is extra important, especially when it comes to seasonal dishes closely associated with the winter holidays. Let's talk about a couple specifics.

DEFROSTING YOUR TURKEY

Allow twenty-four hours for every five pounds of bird defrosting breast side up, in its unopened wrapper, on a tray in the refrigerator. So a twenty pounder, which needs four days to properly defrost, should begin thawing in your fridge sometime on the Sunday before Thanksgiving.

Using the fridge probably is the best method; the worst is thawing your bird on the kitchen counter or anywhere else at room temperature. Don't do it—unless you want to spend the holiday doubled over in the bathroom, which, depending on the family, might not be a bad alternative after all.

Thawing the bird in cold water can be done—but frankly, it's a pain. One method is to completely submerge the still-shrink-wrapped turkey, breast side down, in cold water and then change the water every half hour. This method requires a minimum thawing time of a half hour per pound.

Whatever you do, be sure to consume your fowl entrée within four days of thawing.

Using your Egg Noggin'

To be safe, use only pasteurized eggs in your homemade eggnog, even though many recipes recommend uncooked eggs. If you're working with unpasteurized eggs, cook the yolks lightly with sugar to kill any possible salmonella bacteria.

"What Can We Bring?"

Only you can answer that eternal question from well-meaning guests. And when graciously thanking them in advance, ask that any hot food be sealed in a container for the trip over. On arrival, promptly refrigerate the donated dish—or heat it to 165 degrees Fahrenheit.

Look for a few more general rules of thumb in the checklist at chapter's end.

Vacation Vittles: Getting Away without Getting Sick

Venturing outside the comfort zones of the familiar poses predictable challenges to eating safely. Here are some ideas to chew on from the USDA Food Safety and Inspection Service.[36]

Road Trip!

Hitting the highway means choosing between interstate chain restaurants, mom-and-pop joints and DIY dining. If it's DIY, here are some ideas to keep your meals on wheels safe:

- Bring shelf-stable foods (i.e., canned goods) whenever possible. Perishables—meat, poultry, dairy, salads, etc.—should be held captive in a cooler on ice or frozen gel packs.
- Storing drinks in a separate cooler will keep solid foods chilled longer because the drinks cooler will be opened far more frequently than the food cooler.

---

36 Diane Van, "Keep Food Poisoning from Ruining Your Vacation," *USDA Blog*, United States Department of Agriculture, Aug. 3, 2011, http://blogs.usda.gov.

- If you've got one—and room for it in your vehicle—bring a third cooler devoted solely to carrying each day's food needs so you don't disturb perishables needed for later in the trip.
- Separation is key. Double wrap or use plastic bags for raw meat, poultry or anything with natural juices that could contaminate neighboring foods by mere dripping. We call this the Separation of Chips and Steak, which makes no sense and is present only as a candidate for worst pun of the book.

Destination Dos

Once you arrive, stay safe with some simple tricks of the vacation trade.

CAMPING

Place your cooler in a shady spot—just as you do when parking the car on a hot day. Then cover the cooler with a blanket, tarp or poncho; a white or light-colored cover is best because it reflects the heat from sunlight.[37]

No Time to Get Sloppy

Always wash hands before and after preparing food and use separate plates and utensils for raw and cooked meat (or poultry). Bound for a rustic getaway without running water? Bring soap and water with you. Toss-away wipes are fine for hands but you'll need soap and clean water for the dishes.

BOATING

Be brainy on the briny—don't forget the cooler, and pack plenty of ice. If your food sits out for more than two hours, you've got trouble. And as we've mentioned, if it's ninety degrees Fahrenheit or more outside, the food will only stay safe for a single hour.

---

37 Savvy runners use the same strategy on hot days, which is why they wear white T-shirts or tops to minimize the risk of dehydration.

ON THE BEACH[38]

When you're on the sands, bring just enough food so as to avoid leftovers.

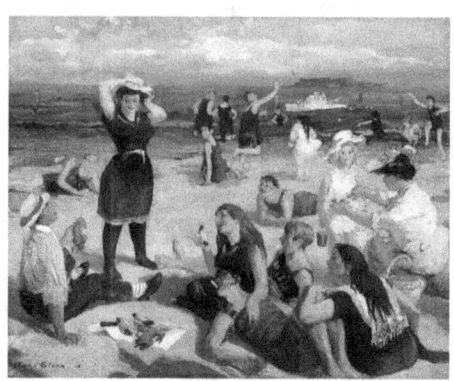

Bury the cooler in the sand, cover with blankets and shade it with an umbrella—you can't be too cautious about keeping things chilled. Check local ordinances beforehand to confirm it's legal to grill on your beach of choice.

RVs AND THE VACATION HOME

If you haven't used your recreational vehicle or visited your vacation home for a while, toss out leftover canned foods from last year; they likely were exposed to freezing temps and ought to be chucked into the next hemisphere.

About the fridge: If it's been unplugged for a year, clean out that sucker before restocking it. Scrub the fridge, food-prep areas and utensils with hot, soapy water.

A Review for You

While food trucks have gone upscale, such rolling kitchens remain just as vulnerable to contamination as they were back in the day. So checking local health laws may help you decide whether that gourmet shish kebab truck is trustworthy. And cleanliness—by truck chefs and by diners too—never goes out of food-prep and -serving style.

Farmers' markets across America are another place where food safety savvy matters. When shopping in the sun, be sure the meats and eggs you buy are properly chilled on-site—and bring a cold-storage bag or container to keep them fresh on the way home.

---

38 Coincidentally, the title of a fine, albeit downbeat, 1959 film about nuclear apocalypse, starring Gregory Peck, Ava Gardner and, in a rare dramatic role, Fred Astaire.

We don't recommend buying milk, cheese or other dairy products from a farmers' market unless you're sure they've been not only chilled but also pasteurized. Ditto for juices and cider, although cold-pressing can be effective in ensuring juice safety.

Wash your hands—disposable towelettes will do—before and after touching produce. And when you get the fruits and veggies home, vigorously rinse them.

When bringing your own food to fairs, festivals and other outdoor events, keep them chilled or warm in the requisite cooler, insulated bag, etc., and be especially careful when it's ninety degrees Fahrenheit or more. At those higher temps, cooked food should be eaten within an hour.

Open-air food vendors should be held to all the standards that restaurants operate under regarding cleanliness, the proper use of utensils and the separation of different foods so that meat or poultry juices don't drip into the salad fixings and the like. Have doubts about the veracity of food vendors? Check them out with a call to your local-government health agency.

Petting zoos are hotbeds of microbial peril. Always wash your hands carefully after contact with animals or their enclosures. If facilities aren't available, try those antibacterial wipes you remembered to bring. You brought them, right?

At holiday time, meal safety begins at home. We covered two widely accepted strategies for safely defrosting your turkey—in the fridge and in water. (The first one's generally better and easier.) We warned you against using unpasteurized eggs in your nog. And we gently advised that you ask guests contributing hot or cold dishes to bring them in temperature-safe containers. Once they're safely at your place, these donated delectables should be either refrigerated or warmed to 165 degrees Fahrenheit.

And for vacationers, we've given you the skinny on how best to pack your road trip repasts so your food is safe while you're camping, boating or chowing down at the beach, in your RV or at that rarely used vacation home.

"What You Can Do" Checklist: Holiday Tips

✓ **Proper cooking temperatures.** Use a thermometer to confirm food has been cooked hot enough to kill bacteria. This means everything—turkey, stuffing, side dishes, even leftovers—should reach at least 165 degrees Fahrenheit. They should be kept north of 140 degrees Fahrenheit during serving; cold foods should be at 40 degrees Fahrenheit.

✓ **Beware of microwave ovens.** They heat unevenly and may not get you to the magic 165 degrees Fahrenheit. In general, the golden rule is to keep hot food hot and cold food cold.

✓ **Love leftovers?** Keep bacteria away by refrigerating leftovers within two hours of meal's end. Store them in shallow containers and don't overstuff the fridge; you need lots of cold air circulating in there. Plus, don't just toss the turkey husk into the fridge. Slice off all remaining meat and pack it in sealed containers or ziplock bags to save space—and to ensure it cools down quickly.

✓ **Wash your hands!** It's the easiest way to prevent or minimize bacterial contamination. And don't cheat. Scrub them with warm water and soap for at least twenty seconds.

✓ **Wash your produce!** Yes, wash even the prepackaged greens in those cellophane bags. A healthy rinsing should do the trick.

✓ **Send Uncle Phil to the living room.** Tell him to join the lively debate there over which football game to watch.[39] Then, barricade the kitchen door—keeping *everybody* out. The holidays fall smack in the middle of cold and flu season. And seriously, nobody wants to try the candied yams once Uncle Phil has swiped his digit through them like a debit card at an ATM. If Phil persists, it's time to break out the alluring appetizers and park them on the coffee table near the partisan screaming over Ohio State vs. Michigan.

---

39 If the Cleveland Browns are playing on Thanksgiving, go with them. Otherwise, you're on your own.

Eight

Taming Tummy Troubles While Traveling

"April in Paris." "When in Rome." "Cleveland Rocks." So many intriguing destinations, so many opportunities to risk your health. When overseas, you naturally want to experience not just the different cultures but also the

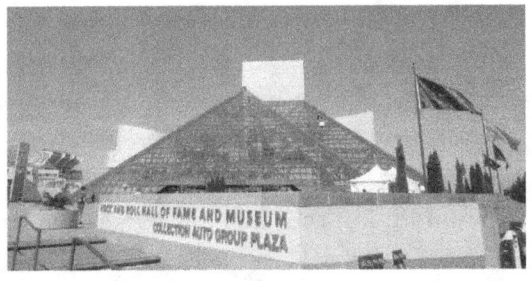

authentic cuisines unavailable at home. But one thing the experimenting epicure doesn't need is a taste of seriously nasty gastrointestinal bugs that can ruin vacations and deliver long-term health horrors—especially in a place with less-than-reliable medical resources or treatment.

No Fish Story

Back in chapter 5, we touched on the fear factors of fish. Stateside, the danger of microbial contamination remains alive and well despite Uncle Sam's approval of irradiation for some seafood. But overseas, mere health threats can morph into dangerous realities. Here are just a few examples.

NONTYPHOIDAL SALMONELLOSIS

Back in chapters one and three, we described at length the gastrointestinal disorder spawned by many serotypes, or versions, of the salmonella bug. Remember that salmonella is transmitted most often through food contaminated with animal feces, but also through direct contact with infected animals or their natural environments. In the United States, an estimated four hundred people die from the illness each year, among the forty-two thousand reported cases. And those are just the *confirmed* cases; the unreported numbers are thought to be much, much higher.

Worldwide, the dangers multiply exponentially. The CDC reports the various strains account for an estimated ninety-four million cases of salmonella's diarrhea and other stomach-turning symptoms. And among those, about 115,000 people a year die from it.[40]

Americans overseas face varying odds of picking up salmonella; it all depends on their destinations. Among those returning home ill, Mexico accounted for 38 percent of the salmonellosis cases. India was second with 9 percent, followed by Jamaica, the Dominican Republic, China and the Bahamas.

SCOMBROID

Scombroid. Just the name sounds evil. In Bali in the winter of 2014, autopsies revealed an Australian tourist and her teenaged daughter died from scombroid after dining on contaminated fish in a restaurant. This common food poisoning is linked to improperly refrigerated or preserved fish plucked from either temperate or tropical waters.

Scombroid is associated with many different kinds of fish; check out the checklist at chapter's end. Symptoms show up within an hour of eating and can easily be mistaken for a bad allergic reaction—flushing of the face with an upper body rash resembling sunburn; severe headache; heart palpitations; itching; fuzzy vision; abdominal cramps; and diarrhea. More serious cases can involve respiratory compromise and malignant arrhythmias.

---

40 Maho Imanishi and Shua J. Chai, "Salmonellosis (Nontyphoidal)," *Yellow Book,* Aug. 1, 2013, http://www.CDC.gov/travel/yellowbook/2014/chapter-3-infectious-diseases-related-to-travel/salmonellosis-nontyphoidal.

Antihistimines often prove effective in treating scombroid. Left untreated, it usually gives up and skulks away within twelve hours. But both Australians suffered from asthma, which seriously complicated their cases. Some experts also speculated the suspect filets may have come from near the fish intestines, which would have delivered a far greater concentration of the scombroid bacteria than other parts of the fish.

Telltale signs? If your fish tastes peppery, sharp, salty or vaguely "bubbly" but otherwise seems normal, watch out. It could be infected, and in many cases neither cooking nor smoking, canning or freezing will kill the histimine—the scombroid toxin.

CIGUATERA

Let's blame ciguatera fish poisoning on Charles Darwin. It's totally unfair, but he'll never know. Darwin's whole survival-of-the-fittest theory[41] seems to fit here since this rather unpleasant food poison comes from eating reef fish contaminated with toxins originating in algae, the teeny organisms growing on or near coral reefs. These mini-marine-meanies, called dinofla-

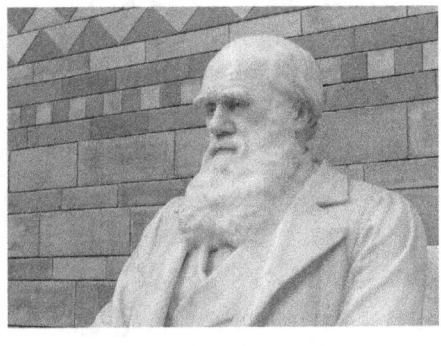

gellates, are devoured by small herbivorous fish. In turn, these fish become lunch for somewhat larger, carnivorous fish, and so on up the food chain to you, me and maybe even Uncle Phil.[42]

Worldwide, more than fifty thousand people a year get ciggy to their stomachs. But that's probably just the tip of the fish head; some experts think ciguatera is vastly underreported and undiagnosed.

Tourists take the brunt—the CDC reports about three of every hundred travelers get sicky from ciggy in "highly endemic areas," usually tropical and

---

41 The cruel irony: Darwin didn't actually coin the phrase "survival of the fittest." That honor belongs to Herbert Spencer (1820–1903), the English philosopher and biologist hugely influenced by Darwinian theory. But blaming Darwin is so much more fun than calling out Spencer.

42 Need a Phil refresher? Revisit chapter 7, under the heading "Healthy Holidays."

subtropical waters. In particular, the Caribbean Sea and the Pacific and Indian Oceans are longtime flashpoints. More recently, danger zones have included the Canary Islands, the eastern Mediterranean and the western Gulf of Mexico.

Ciggy is one nasty bug, producing both classic food poisoning symptoms—nausea, diarrhea, vomiting—and neurological problems resembling chronic fatigue syndrome, including numbness, tingling, joint and muscle pain and dizziness. Sometimes, even stranger sensations develop—such as that your teeth are loose and may fall out or that you've lost the ability to distinguish hot from cold. Don't forget breathing problems, low blood pressure, blurry vision, transient blindness and even a slower heart rate, which can be fatal.

Symptoms begin and fade within hours but sometimes linger for days. In rare cases, the neurological problems hang on, or recur, for months or years.

According to Dr. David Katz, a disease-prevention expert at Yale University, there's no definitive treatment for the neurological problems. He says some patients "find relief in avoiding fish, seafood, alcohol, nuts and nut oils." But Dr. Katz admits that limiting one's diet doesn't necessarily do the job. Most people fully recover—but not until all the residual toxin, which hides in fat tissue, has left the body.[43]

GUILLAIN-BARRÉ SYNDROME

Forget shrunken heads, giant seashells and colorful piñatas. If you're looking to acquire something really exotic on vacation, how about the devastating microbial disorder Guillain-Barré syndrome? Best of all: you don't even have to leave the United States; just explore places like the western part of the border with Mexico.

GBS—mentioned in passing in earlier chapters—is a complication arising from the superbug campylobacter profiled in chapter 3. It tricks the immune system into attacking the body's nerves and can cause paralysis.

In July 2011, at least two dozen GBS cases popped up on both sides of an Arizona stretch of the US-Mexico border. That's a pretty serious outbreak, considering GBS typically affects just one of every hundred thousand

---

43   David L. Katz, MD, "Food Poisoning Caused by Fish," *O: The Oprah Magazine*, March 2009, http://www.oprah.com/health/Food-Poisoning-How-to-Alleviate-Symptoms-of-Ciguatera.

people. Most victims in the border outbreak were left unable to walk; others also experienced upper-body weakness. Officials could formally confirm only four patients infected with campylobacter. But with all the victims' symptoms matching up, the assumption is GBS was the culprit for all.

Campylobacter isn't spread person to person, but rather through undercooked poultry and meat. Keep that in mind, whether you're in Mumbai or Mexico City.

Getting There Is Half the Fun

Even the most fastidious travelers can risk a vacation-ruining illness, or worse, if they don't anticipate the very first threat all air travelers face: the jetliner itself.

- **Smart preparation.** Take immunity-strengthening meds the week before you travel. You need to arm yourself against the inevitable onboard onslaught of bacterial bugs and venal viruses that sidestep even the best efforts of the airlines' crack cleaning crews.
- **Mulling meals at thirty thousand feet.** You probably know that unless you're in first class, many domestic flights have done away with meals altogether, replaced by measly "snacks"—almost always junk food—plus soft drinks or juices.[44] You can settle for those and spend the rest of the flight anxious and hungry. Or you can break down and buy overpriced sandwiches of processed mystery meat and cardboard-like cheese. Don't forget the prefab meals heated in convection ovens—"edibles" you'd never dream of devouring while on terra firma.

Of course, bad-mouthing airline food is the longtime meal ticket of stand-up comedians and the hollow protest of frustrated travelers. Even so, with the march of progress, today's midair meals certainly must be better than back in the day, right?

---

44 Purely on its status as nutritionally bankrupt, alcohol doesn't count here, since its appeal is, well, mostly recreational in nature.

Uh, well…

In 2012, the ABC News program *20/20* reported on more than fifteen hundred health violations the FDA found at airline food facilities during the previous four years. The findings at one subcontractor's kitchen were typical: the presence of vermin, dirty cooking areas, old or moldy ingredients and poor hygiene by employees and others.

Two years earlier, the FDA discovered numerous such facilities were storing food at the wrong temperatures and cooking on dirty equipment operated by employees with rather nasty ideas about hygiene. Then there were the cockroaches. And the flies. And the mice.

Do these horrors typically produce onboard gross outs? The airlines usually say no, but ponderous problems popped up at least twice in 2012 alone. In April that year, an Australian woman on an international flight noticed an unusual texture in the trail mix she purchased on that flight. Seems it was maggots. Other packets of the same snack were similarly swarming with fly larvae.

In July that year on a flight into Toronto, a passenger found a sewing needle. Not in an etui or a pincushion. In his *sandwich*. Alas, not a stitch of thread in sight, either.

The smart solution, part I. Eat hearty before heading for the airport. Taking an early morning flight? Indulge yourself with a megabreakfast, a healthy habit to have anyway. It'll fuel you for the flight and ground those fitful urges to snack on airport (and airline) junk food.

The smart solution, part II. If you didn't eat before leaving home, bringing your own food may be the best alternative, assuming you can get it past the Transportation Security Administration (TSA) agents. Which shouldn't be a problem, if it's dry food that fits in a carry-on bag. We're talking about benign, healthful goodies such as nuts and trail mix, granola, cereal, dried fruit, even immunity-boosting raw fruit and veggies. Another immune system ally is yogurt, *if you can get it past security*.[45] You'll need every available nutritional defense against other passengers sneezing and wheezing from colds, flu and who knows what.

---

45 Another challenge with yogurt, besides its near-liquid nature, is keeping it cold. As of 2014, the Transportation Security Administration hadn't prohibited gel-filled cold packs as carry-on items. But the TSA periodically revises its rules, so it's best to check before you travel.

And don't get a false sense of security by assuming sick seniors or coughing kids are sitting far enough away from you. Thanks to the miracle of recirculating cabin air, you're guaranteed a democratic, share-the-misery experience while jetting off to that heartfelt reunion with Uncle Phil.

The smart solution, part III. If the fates conspire to stick you with airline food, go for the healthiest available choices—raw foods including fruit or leafy green salads, nuts (instead of chips, crackers or pretzels) and, in lieu of soda, healthful juices like orange and apple.

Drown your doubts in H$_2$O. When traveling, you can't hydrate too much. Especially in the air, when your body is adapting to high altitudes and there's a relative lack of mobility for hours. While you can't legally bring plastic water bottles past airport security, you can buy water (yes, for a premium price) inside the terminal while en route to the gate. The other option is to nag, pester and annoy the flight attendants for water refills throughout the flight. Besides, friendly badgering just might be more entertaining than many in-flight movies, like, for example, *The Wiggles Meet the Teletubbies in Outer Space.*

Okay, I'm Here and I'm Hungry—Now What?

You've landed far from home and you're famished. What can you eat that's safe—and what will make you sorry? Here are some guidelines.

Watch the water. In countries like Mexico, foreign visitors often end up doubled over. You know: "Montezuma's revenge"—the now politically incorrect phrase referring to the stomach-turning effects of parasites found in Mexican drinking water.[46] Those who grow up with it develop immunity to those parasites. But Americans and other visitors fall victim because their bodies are only familiar with, and thus tolerant of, the parasites basking in the tap water back home.

So beware of fruit shakes and any beverages mixed with water. Even ice should be shunned since it likely consists of unpurified water. Don't risk a drink from a street vendor unless you're certain it contains purified water. The

---

46 In February 1979, then president Jimmy Carter, on a state visit to Mexico, made an offhand wisecrack about "Montezuma's revenge" to his Mexican counterpart, José López Portillo. Mexico's leader was highly offended and Carter's remark touched off a diplomatic controversy.

safest method is to pick only tourist-oriented eateries—a drag for the more adventurous traveler—where purified water is indicated clearly on the menu.

Safe water sources. Don't despair—there's plenty of potable water available on vacation:

- Bring local water to a rolling boil to kill most microorganisms.
- Bottled water is usually reliable, but check that the seal is unbroken for assurance the bottle hasn't been refilled from the tap.
- Purified water is plentiful wherever you travel if you bring your own portable purifier. Effective, handheld systems are available. The catch: these can cost up to $150.
- You can chemically disinfect water by dropping iodine-based tablets into it before drinking. But follow instructions to the letter and know the tablets are unreliable if your water appears cloudy or is contaminated with organic material—soil, leafy matter or, ahem, unmentionable stuff.

Otherwise, trust your inner cynic and assume all other water sources are contaminated. Don't even brush your teeth in uncertain waters; use the bottled variety instead.

Heat kills. Got nagging doubts about that plateful of food in front of you? How long, you wonder, has the meat, poultry or fish been sitting around? How was it handled? Regardless of how your protein was prepared—fried, boiled, broiled, baked, broasted, whatever—make sure your hosts turn up the heat high enough to kill germs. (Unless it's the impervious-to-heat scombroid toxin, histimine.) Still nervous? As you chew the fat with dining companions, eschew the meat altogether—it will turn bad faster than any vegetable.

Yogurt: the "good" bacteria. So what's the difference between yogurt and Los Angeles? Yogurt has an active culture. (Insert rim shot, canned laughter.)

Sure, the gag's as lame now as it was in 1983. Or 1883. The point is that yogurt contains probiotics (literally, "for life"), the "good" bacteria that actually promote health.[47] Some of these good-guy microbes adjust the microflora, or natural balance of organisms, in the intestines. Others aid digestion and the

---

47 More on probiotics just ahead in chapter 9.

immune system. But not all yogurt products have probiotics, so make sure the label confirms that "live and active cultures" are indeed inside.

Low-fly zone. Remember Renfield from the 1930 Universal Pictures classic *Dracula*? Driven insane by the count, Renfield becomes obsessed with eating flies. We're not advocating flies as an entrée, despite the selling point they're fat- and cholesterol-free—the little buzzers can carry disease. But do pay attention to the fly population when you consider food from a street vendor or a sit-down restaurant. If the flies are few, that's a good sign. If they're plentiful, watch out.

Turnover (not of the apple variety). The faster the turnover of food, the likelier it's fresh and safe. It stands to reason the longer food sits around—on a grill, in a pan or otherwise exposed to the elements—the greater chance it will draw bacteria. Equally intuitive is the notion that the quicker a dish is sold and replaced with freshly cooked food, the likelier it's pretty safe to eat—and that its popularity means it's tasty.

Find your inner fussbudget. Don't be afraid to give the once-over to your drinking glass and silverware. Clean them with a napkin (and bottled or purified water) if necessary. And since drinking glasses cleaned with unpurified local water can be dangerous, consider drinking directly from a bottle or can.

You, too, can be a-peelin'. Regarding fruits and vegetables, go for those you can peel yourself—bananas, papayas, avocados and so on. Try to avoid lettuce or anything with a skin (like a tomato) because it might have been washed with tainted water. If you can't avoid risky produce, insist it be washed in purified and slightly chlorinated water.

Trust no one. Be wary of food safety even if you're traveling on an organized (i.e., packaged) tour. Don't assume that because travel "experts" made the arrangements, you'll be eating safely everywhere. Travel tours can't guarantee all proper safety precautions will be followed along the way. Something as simple as a dirty utensil can turn a trek through Asia into a trip to bountiful nausea.

A Review for You

International travel is no fun when you're writhing in agony from food-borne illness. In this chapter, we looked at illnesses you could face in a foreign country. Some fish are particular carriers of bad-news bugs:

- **Nontyphoidal salmonellosis** can be responsible for diarrhea, abdominal cramps and fever lasting as long as a week. Mexico has the dubious distinction of leading the pack, generating 38 percent of salmonellosis cases among all American tourists. India is a distant second with 9 percent. Other hot spots include Jamaica, the Dominican Republic, China and the Bahamas.

- **Scombroid poisoning** is linked to poor refrigeration or improper preservation of fish. While many symptoms—including flushed face, severe upper-body rash and headache—often resolve within twelve hours, serious cases can be life-threatening. Among telltale signs of contamination: fish with a peppery, sharp, salty or "bubbly" taste. Now the really bad news: neither cooking nor smoking, canning or freezing will kill the scombroid toxin.

- **Ciguatera food poisoning** is traced to algae growing on or near coral reefs. Tourists account for most victims, who acquire it primarily in tropical and subtropical areas. Worst-hit regions include the Caribbean, the Pacific and Indian Oceans, the Canary Islands, the eastern Mediterranean and the western Gulf of Mexico. Ciguatera presents classic food poisoning symptoms (nausea, diarrhea, etc.), plus symptoms reminiscent of chronic fatigue syndrome (numbness, joint pain and others). Additional effects include vision loss, a sense of loose teeth and difficulty discerning between hot and cold. Most people recover quickly, but some fatalities are reported, and for survivors of severe cases, the scarier symptoms can hang on for years.

- **Guillain-Barré syndrome**, as we discussed earlier, is a complication of the superbug campylobacter. It messes with the immune system and can cause paralysis. GBS is spread via undercooked poultry and meat, so make sure your vacation protein gets fully cooked.

- **Water, water everywhere,** yet you're often just a gulp away from gastrointestinal bedlam. While visiting lands of troubled waters, be resolute: avoid ice, and be wary of drinks from street vendors. Sip directly from cans or bottles—your drinking glass may have been washed with unpurified water. Clutch bottled water to your bosom—but beware of broken seals, a sign the bottle was refilled with unclean tap water. Bring along your own hand-held water pour-through purifying system; chemically disinfect water with iodine tablets, although they're not always reliable; or boil your water to rid it of illness-bearing bacteria. Contaminated water can also undo you when swallowed or inhaled while swimming, bathing or showering. So let's be careful out there.

"What You Can Do" Checklist: Travel Tactics

THE CDC IS YOUR FRIEND

Before you leave home, check the Centers for Disease Control's website for an excellent roundup of current health information on just about any destination in the world. The CDC also offers the following.

- ✓ **Travel notices.** The CDC warns you about any current problems or issues at specific destinations, using a three-level format: Watch Level 1 means to practice your usual precautions; Alert Level 2 urges "enhanced" precautions; and Warning Level 3 means "Avoid nonessential travel"—roughly translated from the bureaucratese as "Just stay away."
- ✓ **Pretravel planning.** This includes advice about which vaccines or medicines to get *before* leaving and can help you locate travel clinics in the United States that specialize in travel medicine.
- ✓ **Disease directory.** The CDC lists specific diseases you could confront at your destination(s).
- ✓ **The Yellow Book.** Find out about this CDC informational travel guide published every other year by Oxford University Press. It's an excellent reference on health risks around the world and available in hard copy or as a smartphone app.

JUST SAY "NAH"
Foods to avoid:

- ✓ Uncooked or undercooked food, especially seafood and eggs
- ✓ Salads or fruits and veggies you can't peel
- ✓ Ice cream
- ✓ Unpasteurized dairy products (don't assume any are pasteurized)
- ✓ Dishes that need a lot of food handling during preparation

RISKY FISHNESS
Beware the following swimmers and their potential to infect.

Scombroid	✓ Amberjack
	✓ Anchovy
	✓ Bluefish
	✓ Herring
	✓ Mackerel
	✓ Sardine
	✓ Mahimahi
	✓ Marlin
	✓ Tuna
Ciguatera	✓ Barracuda
	✓ Grouper
	✓ Mackerel
	✓ Moray eel
	✓ Parrot fish
	✓ Red snapper
	✓ Sea bass
	✓ Sturgeon

THE OLDEST TRICK IN THE BOOK

Why, it's hand washing, of course. Remember to always, always, *always* scrub them.

✓ Wash with soap and hot running water, using the 20/20 rule: twenty seconds soaping up and rinsing off, twenty seconds drying with a clean towel. The bonus: You just might avoid more colds and flu too.

✓ Use disposable wipes or alcohol-based gels if clean water isn't available.

✓ Wash hands after visiting the toilet.

✓ Wash hands before and after meals.

✓ Wash hands whenever you've clutched oft-touched transportation surfaces such as train and bus railings. The fact is, you can't wash your hands too much while traveling.

Nine

W e're now eight jam-packed chapters in—and yet we've provided precious little practical advice on coping with food poisoning. Your wait is over. Most of this chapter is common sense stuff, but that doesn't diminish its importance, especially when you're in dire distress.

A Good Excuse to Start Drinking

In most routine cases of food poisoning, you'll likely recover within twelve to forty-eight hours. Don't count on your doctor prescribing anything—antibiotics, for example—because most cases don't require it and they wouldn't help anyway.

In routine situations, strategy number one—pulled directly from the "D" file[48]—goes without saying: get plenty of rest. Staying off your feet really helps you bounce back faster. Besides, food poisoning may be the best excuse ever for binge viewing that hip cable series you never found time to watch.[49]

---

48 As in "Duh."

49 While still in the vomit or diarrheal stage, it's probably best to avoid *The Walking Dead*. Jus' sayin'.

The next priority: guard against dehydration. You really can't drink too much water (or other clear liquids) to replenish the minerals and fluids lost to diarrhea and vomiting. Start with small sips and build up from there.

If diarrhea and vomiting hang on more than twenty-four hours, you'll need an oral rehydration solution. Oral rehydration liquids (Pedialyte, for example) and powders, the latter mixed with water, are widely available at pharmacies. Or make your own by dissolving into 4 1/4 cups (1 liter) of water a half teaspoon of salt, a half teaspoon of baking soda and 4 tablespoons of sugar.

If you already happen to be taking a diuretic, ask a medical professional if you should discontinue taking it during the illness-inspired diarrhea. But don't change or stop taking any of your regular meds before checking with your doctor's office.

Over-the-counter diarrhea treatments are available at the pharmacy. But again, let common sense prevail: first check with your doctor or healthcare provider. And especially avoid them if the diarrhea is bloody or severe or if you have a fever.

Who You Gonna Call?

If you're seriously dehydrated or suspect your food poisoning is due to seafood, mushrooms or botulism, don't hesitate: Call 911.

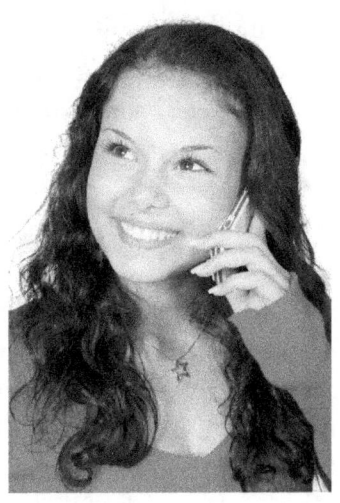

Otherwise, you probably won't need to consult a doctor except in these urgent cases:

- Call if the diarrhea lasts more than three days, or two days in a child or infant.
- Call if your fever surpasses 101°F (or if a child's fever is at least 100.4°F) when accompanied by diarrhea.
- Call if diarrhea occurs after eating seafood or mushrooms.
- Call if the diarrhea is bloody or dark or if it contains pus.
- If diarrhea is accompanied by vomiting that prevents you from keeping liquids down, 911 will likely direct you to the hospital for intravenous fluids.

- Get help for severe dehydration, the symptoms of which include dry mouth, dizziness, fatigue, a drop in urination or an increase in either heart rate or breathing rate.
- Call for help if a child has been vomiting for at least twelve hours.
- Anyone caring for an infant age three months or younger should call for medical advice immediately if the infant begins vomiting or has diarrhea.

I Know I Should Eat Something

Mom was right—when you're sick, you can't just go on eating anything you want, not if you hope to bounce back in a day or two. So until the vomiting spells are over, it's no big deal, nutritionally speaking, to walk on eggshells around your stomach. If temptation calls, activate that inner-discipline chip and run like the wind from solid foods.

Once the heaving halts, eat light and bland—the kind of stuff you might snub under normal circumstances. And actually, while crawling your way back from food poisoning, even the most normally adventurous gastronome will find crackers, bananas, rice or bread irresistible delicacies.

Even when you're healthy, we don't recommend fried or greasy foods. But be absolutely sure to shun them while struggling with nausea and vomiting. The same goes for spicy stuff and sweets too.

Good News and Less-Than-Good News

First, the good news: *Conventional* wisdom holds that hardly anybody dies from bacterial food poisoning—at least hardly anybody who is otherwise healthy.

Now the not-so-good news: There may be a major undercounting of deaths triggered by food bugs—because food poisoning may hasten deaths in those people with immune systems already compromised by other serious illnesses. And as we've noted, gastrointestinal ailments can also have long-term, serious effects that can devastate your quality of life.

A Review for You

It's no secret food poisoning is a pretty lousy experience, but you can mitigate the misery with common sense approaches including resting, drinking lots of clear liquids, staying (mostly) away from solid food and sticking to the blandly safe "sick foods." Which leads us to…

"What You Can Do" Checklist: "Sick Food"

MIGHTY-SAFE EATIN'

Sure, for those suffering from a food-borne illness, mealtime is no picnic. Here are some tried-and-true "sick foods" benign enough to help until you feel free of fever, rebound from regurgitation and declare victory over vomiting:

- ✓ Clear broths and soup
- ✓ Fruit juices
- ✓ Water (you can't drink too much of it)
- ✓ Flat ginger ale
- ✓ Soft fruits and vegetables (cooked carrots, for example)
- ✓ Gelatin
- ✓ Frozen fruit pops
- ✓ Congee, the Chinese version of gooey, soft, creamy rice porridge. (Congee has many variations throughout Asia, but all begin with rice and a lot of liquid—usually water—plus a bit of salt. It can be sweetened by adding fruit, particularly pears and apples. Congee can be prepared on the stovetop, in a slow cooker or in a rice cooker. In Japan, it's called *okayu*, while for Koreans and Thais it's *juk* and *jok*, respectively—and that's no joke.)

And there's the "BRAT diet," a simple guide to get you through those bacterial belly battles:

✓ **B**ananas, good for restoring potassium lost to vomiting
✓ **R**ice (think congee) or rice pudding
✓ **A**pplesauce, to help settle your stomach
✓ **T**oast (dry) or crackers

DON'T EVEN THINK ABOUT IT

Besides the aforementioned fried, greasy and spicy items, stay away from foods high in the following:

✓ Fat
✓ Dairy
✓ Fiber

Ten

The Secret to a Clean-Living Diet? Trust Good Old Auntie Inflammatory

A long time ago, in a world far different from today, President Franklin Roosevelt famously declared that a certain late-autumn date would "live in infamy."[50] If FDR lived today, he could rightfully claim humanity now lives with *inflammy*, that is, inflammation.

No, not the swollen, painful, discolored, red-hot-thumb kind you get showing off your carpentry skills. We mean *invisible* inflammation—the kind quietly spreading, needlessly and wildly, inside the body.

Chronic inflammation is considered the root of many age-related health scourges such as cardiovascular disease and cancer, neurodegenerative tragedies including Alzheimer's and other

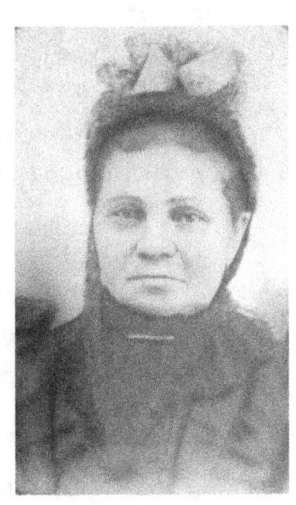

Dear old Auntie Inflammatory. She tried to tell us, but we were immune to her warnings.

---

50 In FDR's December 8, 1941, appearance before Congress, the president requested a declaration of war following the previous day's massive Japanese attack on Pearl Harbor, Hawaii, which he labeled "a date which will live in infamy."

dementias, Parkinson's and Huntington's diseases, autoimmune disorders (especially rheumatoid arthritis) and other illnesses.

Under normal circumstances, inflammation is a regular, important and welcome weapon in the immune system's biologic arsenal of healing responses to injuries or attack, microbial or otherwise. And like the American body politic, the human body has built-in checks and balances to keep inflammation from overdoing its job and going haywire. But if those protections fail, and inflammation spreads beyond a damaged area, even at imperceptibly low levels, it eventually shreds the body's autoimmune defenses by actually promoting and producing disease.

So what influences a person's inflammatory tendencies? Besides genetics, there's contact with environmental toxins, secondhand smoke and stress. But—stem cell research aside—can anyone control their own genetic blueprint? And who can swear they've completely avoided exposure or proximity to environmental poisons? Or to cigarette smoke, for that matter?

Oh, and if you've somehow dodged stress all your life, we really want to meet you.

There is, however, one proven way you can wield enormous control over losing your immune system's mojo. C'mon, don't be coy—you know what we mean.

You have the power to decide what you want to eat, how you like it prepared and how best to choose foods that both promote health and provide anti-inflammatory fuel for your immune system.

A Diet to Help You Live without Inflammation

Dr. Andrew Weil, the Harvard-trained holistic physician known for integrative medicine,[51] has long advocated an anti-inflammatory diet. "You want to include as much fresh food as possible," he told an audience in a video posted to his website. "I think the main rule—and I must say if I could summarize

---

51 Integrative medicine seeks to combine alternative therapies with conventional treatments.

everything I know about nutrition in one sentence, it would be, 'Stop eating refined, processed and manufactured food.' It's that simple."[52]

He's right. No question that prefab foods—highly processed and/or refined stuff, from sugar to packaged luncheon meats to cookies and way beyond—certainly are convenient. But you pay a devastating price for that ease of use because they're also stripped of antioxidants and critical probiotics—"good bacteria"—your body needs to control inflammation.

Dr. Weil's simple nutrition rule forces the question, "Well, just what *can* I eat that's safe, healthful, wholesome, actually tastes good—and won't make me feel like a rabbit nibbling on lettuce and feigning fulfillment?"

The answer lies with sweet old Auntie Inflammatory, the diet sometimes known as the clean-living regimen.[53] It's akin to the familiar heart-healthy Mediterranean diet known for the generous use of olive oil in cooking, red wine, servings of fresh fruits and veggies, fish, whole grains, nuts and legumes and for minimizing meats, sweets, poultry and dairy.

Generally, the clean-living (anti-inflammatory) diet follows some basic rules:

- **Modified food? File under "D" for *duh*.** Remember Dr. Weil's rule? It bears repeating: *Cut refined, processed and manufactured food out of your life.* Be ruthless. Dump anything created in a food-conglomerate lab devised by well-meaning food scientists simply obeying corporate marching orders to create composite edibles capable of 156-year shelf lives.
- Having any doubts about just what constitutes processed food? Easy—it's *anything with a label*, that is, anything requiring *more than a single ingredient to make.* This especially includes refined sugar, which for many people won't be easy to quit but will make a sweet world of difference once you give it the heave-ho.

---

52 "Why Should We Eat an Anti-Inflammatory Diet?" https://www.drweil.com/drw/u/PAG00361/anti-inflammatory-food-pyramid.html.

53 Also "eating clean," "eat clean," "whole food" and other, similar sounding diet names.

- **Eat whole foods.** Focus on things left unaltered while in the test lab or the food factory—stuff straight from the farm, unmessed with by Dr. Frankenstein–style food science. Think of a whole food as a handmade wooden bookcase designed and built by a master craftsman (nature), as opposed to a shaky, mass-produced particleboard bookcase with a flimsy wood-veneer exterior that splits apart soon after assembly.
- The purity of some whole foods is exemplified in staples such as whole fruits, veggies, unsalted nuts, seeds and grains. Less obvious examples, like grass-fed and free-range meats and low-fat dairy products, require that you pay attention to packaging.
- **More and smaller meals.** Transition to five or six littler meals spread throughout the day. This will kick your metabolism up and make it easier to skip those nutritionally bankrupt snacks you'd otherwise wolf down.
- **Do it yourself.** Cook. Make your meals from scratch. Clean, whole foods are not just healthier, they're often simple to prepare.
- **Bring back balance.** Your meals should make common sense combinations—protein with carbs, for example, or carbs with fat. Believe it or not, better balance will kill your between-meal hunger attacks and also provide fuel to keep you going, thanks to greater metabolic efficiency.

Auntie Inflammatory's Clean-Livin' Food List

Okay, so you're sold on driving the highway to Clean Livin'. But where's the onramp? We're saving a comprehensive list of healing, healthful herbs and spices for the checklist at chapter's end. First, here's a foodie road map to increased immunity and clean cooking—one that doesn't sacrifice flavor:

- **Cooked Asian mushrooms. Unlimited servings.** Any fun guy will tell you fungi can work wonders on your immune system. In many Asian cultures, mushrooms are regarded equally as fine food and effective herbal remedies. Closer to home, the American Cancer Society reports that in animal studies, the chemical compounds in shiitake mushrooms have shown antitumor (cancer-fighting), cholesterol-lowering (cardiovascular) and virus-inhibiting properties. (The ACS, however, does add that clinical studies are needed to see if such health benefits extend to humans.[54]) But a couple caveats: never eat mushrooms raw, and don't overdo it on two popular button varieties—crimini (brown) 'shrooms and their more mature relative, the portobello. Gorging on these two can generate enough uric acid in your system to give you gout and kidney stones. On the other hand, it's safe to freely indulge in cooked Asian mushroom varieties including these:

- o **Shiitake**
- o **Enokidake**
- o **Maitake**
- o **Oyster mushrooms**

- **Healthful fats. Two to three servings a day.** Like "military intelligence," "paid volunteer" or "friendly takeover," the phrase "healthful fats" sounds like an oxymoron—until you consider that a fair number of cooking oils, nuts, seeds and other foods and ingredients are bursting with healthful monounsaturated and/or omega-3 fats. One serving equals a tablespoon of oil, two walnuts, a tablespoon of flaxseed or an ounce of avocado. Candidates for your consideration:

  - o **Extra-virgin olive oil or expeller-pressed canola oil,** used in cooking
  - o The aforementioned **walnuts, avocado and freshly ground flaxseed**
  - o **Hemp seeds**
  - o **Cold-water fish**

---

54 Reported on Cancer.org, accessed March 19, 2015, http://www.cancer.org/treatment/treatmentsandsideeffects/complementaryandalternativemedicine/dietandnutrition/shiitake-mushroom.

- ○ **Omega-3–enriched eggs**
- ○ **Whole soy foods** (see below for details)
- ○ **Organic, expeller-pressed, high-oleic sunflower or safflower oils**
- ○ **Walnut or hazelnut oils,** with salads
- ○ **Dark-roasted sesame oil**, for seasoning soups and stir-fries

- **Vegetables. Four to eight servings daily.** Actually, you can enjoy unlimited quantities of vegetables, so don't say you're hungry. Like their
  fruity brethren, veggies just gush antioxidant and anti-inflammatory flavonoids and carotenoids. A serving is the equivalent of either one cup raw (salad greens, etc.) or a half cup of other vegetables served any way you like—cooked,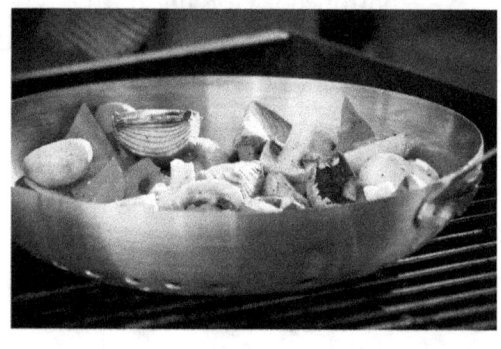
  raw, even liquefied into juice. Go for a variety of colors, and again, organic is best:

- ○ **Spinach**
- ○ **Collard greens**
- ○ **Kale**
- ○ **Swiss chard**
- ○ **Broccoli**
- ○ **Cabbage**
- ○ **Brussels sprouts**
- ○ **Bok choy**
- ○ **Cauliflower**
- ○ **Carrots**
- ○ **Beets**
- ○ **Onions**

- o **Peas**[55]
- o **Squash**
- o **Sea vegetables**
- o **Raw salad greens (washed)**

- **Whole and intact grains. Three to four servings each day.** Because whole grains—grains intact or in large chunks—mitigate the frequency of blood-sugar spikes, you'll gain a measure of protection from inflammation. Serving size: a half cup of cooked grains. Unfortunately, neither whole wheat bread nor other foods fashioned from flour fit here. Those foods that do include these:

  - o **Brown, basmati and wild rice**
  - o **Buckwheat**
  - o **Barley**
  - o **Quinoa,** the seed often considered a whole grain, frequently prepared and served like rice
  - o **Groats,** hulled kernels of whole cereal grains such as oat, wheat and rye
  - o **Steel-cut oats**
  - o **Amaranth,** a grain popular with the Aztecs and available mostly at health-food stores, packed with nutrients, especially trace metals (must be cooked for human consumption)
  - o **Freekeh (frikeh),** a Middle Eastern cereal derived from roasted green wheat, high in fiber and with a low glycemic index, which makes it helpful in managing diabetes
  - o **Millet,** a grain mix most widely available in a hulled variety that, when prepared, is creamy, like mashed potatoes, goes well with many meals and, like amaranth, is loaded with important metals

- **Fruits. Three to four servings daily.** A treasure trove of flavonoids and carotenoids, fruit's naturally occurring plant pigments cut the

---

55 Actually a legume. So sue us.

risks of cancer, heart disease and stroke. Frozen or fresh (in season) are fine; organic is best.

Serving size: a medium piece of fruit, or a half cup of cut-up or chopped fruit. With dried fruit, a serving is just a quarter cup. Warning: fruit has significant sugar content, so if you're overweight, obese, either prediabetic or diabetic or if you have metabolic syndrome,[56] stick with no more than two fruit servings a day and avoid fruit juice and dried fruits. The following are among the best bets:

- **Raspberries**
- **Blueberries**
- **Strawberries**
- **Blackberries**
- **Nectarines**
- **Oranges**
- **Pink grapefruit**
- **Red grapes**
- **Plums**
- **Pomegranates**
- **Cherries**
- **Apples**
- **Pears**
- **Peaches**

- **Beans and legumes. One to two servings daily.** Did you spring from bed this morning and think, "Gosh! I've just *gotta* find something full of folic acid, maxed out with magnesium, packin' potassium and stuffed with soluble fiber, protein and carbs"? Read no further. Beans and legumes are the answer.[57] Serving size: a half cup, cooked whole. You can also puree beans and legumes into terrific spreads, which

56 A group of health risk factors. When two or more occur together, there's a progressive increase in the risk of heart disease, diabetes and stroke. The individual risk factors include increased blood pressure, high blood sugar, excess body fat around the waist and abnormal cholesterol levels.

57 Don't let this get out, but technically speaking, beans, like peas, are legumes too.

explains why an otherwise wussy, sad-sack legume like the lowly chickpea,[58] with the help of a food processor, seasonings and some talented marketing and PR personnel, can be magically transformed into hummus, among the great spreads of the world.

o **Anasazi beans**
o **Adzuki beans**
o **Black beans**
o **Chickpeas,** a.k.a. **garbanzo beans**
o **Black-eyed peas**
o **Lentils**

- **Tea. Two to four cups a day.** Certain teas are natural antioxidants, thanks to catechins, crystalline flavonoid compounds sworn to be loyal to the anti-inflammy cause. Seek out high-quality varieties of white, green and oolong teas.
- **Whole soy foods. One to two servings a day.** These cancer-hatin' goodies with antioxidant isoflavones are the real deal. Don't be fooled by "unwhole" fractionated (i.e., processed) soy foods like soy protein powders and pretend meats fashioned from soy isolate. Try these single servings: a half cup of either tofu, tempeh or cooked edamame; a cup of soy milk; or an ounce of soy nuts. *Important note: Only consume organic soy products!* Insist upon foods with (or of) real soy, not the genetically modified stuff.
- **Red wine (optional). One to two glasses a day.** For years we've heard of its antioxidant power, thanks to the presence of resveratrol. Now, however, some experts have their doubts.[59] If you choose not to share

---

58 A.k.a. garbanzo bean.

59 [62] An eleven-year study of nearly eight hundred elderly Italians cast doubt on long-held claims that resveratrol, a chemical found in red wine, grapes, certain berries and dark chocolate, has health-enhancing and life-extending properties due to antioxidant, anti-inflammatory and anti-cancer properties. Instead, the study found no measurable effect on health and longevity. It was published May 12, 2014, in *JAMA Internal Medicine*. More information is available at http://archinte.jamanetwork.com/article.aspx?articleid=1868537.

in the doubt, organic red wine is best. Merlot, for example, can be a solid source of resveratrol, depending on growing conditions, grape quality and winemaking procedures.

- **Multivitamin/multimineral supplements. Daily.** Supplements can fill in micronutrient gaps in your diet. Look for those with antioxidants including vitamins C and E, mixed carotenoids, selenium, the energy-generating coenzyme Q10, up to three grams of a molecularly distilled fish oil and 2,000 IU of vitamin D$_3$.
- **Tonic herbs (adaptogens).** These help build energy and immunity, producing resistance to, and insulating the body from, the nasty effects of physiological stresses. Adaptogens can be traced back thousands of years to early use in Chinese herbal medicine. Modern studies began in the late 1940s. One of the better adaptogens, holy basil, also called tulsi, is an excellent anti-inflammatory and helps keep your system on an even keel by modulating biochemicals tied to stress responses, especially including cortisol, a steroid hormone associated with belly fat. Just as you take daily vitamins, you should consider taking adaptogens. More on the multitalented holy basil (tulsi) in the checklist at chapter's end.
- **Fish and seafood. Two to six servings weekly.** These mercenaries in the war against inflammation are crammed with inflammation-fightin' omega-3 fats. Your servings, incidentally, should each weigh in at four ounces. The best swimmers to consider are these:

  o **Salmon, sockeye in particular.** You'll need the right kind of salmon to gain the antioxidant benefits, and that usually means wild salmon from Alaskan waters. *(Warning: stern lecture begins here.)* Avoid like the plague the farm-raised salmon so ubiquitous in stores today—unless, of course, you crave its stratospheric levels (up to ten times more than in wild salmon) of cancer-causing toxins. *(Lecture continues. Sit up straight and stop talking.)* Not to mention the traces of antibiotics and other drugs the poor guys ingested during brief, unhappy lives spent flopping around the jam-packed, cruelly cramped fish farms where they were specifically bred solely for human consumption. Farmed salmon have fewer omega fatty acids and contain less protein than their wild cousins. *(Lecture continues. Pay attention. There will be a quiz.)* Even worse, the entire salmon-farming trade is ecologically disastrous, actually posing a threat to the ocean's natural resources. So avoid buying farmed salmon. When dining out, always ask your waiter the source of the salmon you're considering. *(Okay, lecture over. Be ready for midterms next week.)*

- ○ **Herring**
- ○ **Sardines**
- ○ **Black cod,** sometimes called **sablefish**

Not a seafarin' fish fan? You can still get the omega-3 fatty acids fish provide from a daily, molecularly distilled fish oil supplement that includes fatty acids EPA and DHA. Your dose: two to three grams a day.

- • **Pasta al dente. Two to three servings a week.** Ever undercooked pasta and thought you'd hopelessly screwed it up? Relax—you've actually done yourself a favor. When noodles are still a bit firm, you've actually prepared them "al dente," Italian for "to the tooth." Compared to soft pasta, al dente pasta enjoys a lower, healthier position on the glycemic index, which measures carbs and their effect on blood sugar. Such low glycemic-load carbs help control jumps in blood glucose levels. But why are you still reading this when all you care about is the list of al dentables?

- ○ **Organic pasta**
- ○ **Rice noodles**
- ○ **Bean-thread noodles**
- ○ **Japanese udon and soba noodles,** or other comparable pastas that are part whole wheat and part buckwheat

- **Alternate proteins. One to two servings a week.** In general, aim for more of a plant-based diet, but good protein sources are listed below. A serving equals any one of the following: an ounce of cheese; an eight-ounce serving of dairy; an egg; or three ounces of cooked poultry or skinless meat. These are among your healthiest choices:

  o **Natural cheeses** such as **Emmental** (named for the Swiss region where it originated), **Jarlsberg** and real **Parmesan,** not the grated stuff in a paper can
  o **Natural yogurt**
  o **Omega-3–enriched eggs** from hens raised on a flax-enriched diet
  o **Organic eggs** from free-range chickens
  o **Grass-fed lean meats**
  o **Organic, cage-free, skinned poultry**

- **Healthful sweets. Sparingly. On rare occasion. Don't push it.** Dark chocolate, for one, is nice. Maybe even swell—apologies to dear old Auntie Inflammatory—because its antioxidants snap up those pesky free radicals (remember them?) implicated in heart disease. But don't go crazy; there's decided divergence in the medical community over whether dark's powers (not unlike resveratrol) are strong enough to be real…or mostly a sweet dream.

Jump-Starting That Old Immune System of Yours

The sad fact is inflammation has been undercutting the human autoimmune system for a long time. There are various theories meant to account for this, including one that posits we live in a too-clean society.[60]

It's important to note there are easy dietary choices and changes available to boost your immune system's effectiveness. The key is getting critically needed probiotics—remember the "good bacteria"?—back where they're needed.

---

60 We considered placing a Miley Cyrus joke here, but thought the better of it.

Fermenting a Revolution: Power to the Pickle!

Among options to jump-start that old autoimmune system is the ancient food art of fermentation.

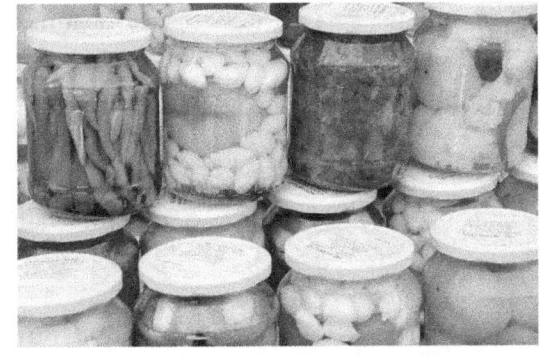

You perked up at "fermentation," didn't you? Sorry, but we're not prescribing brewskis. Wellness experts, however, do get excited over fermented *foods*, believing they pack the gut ("digestive tract" in polite society) with probiotic "good" bacteria that aid the body in various ways, including boosting immunity.

You remember fermentation from high school chemistry or maybe that wine-tasting weekend in Napa Valley? If not, here's a refresher:

Fermentation—or "culturing"—is the chemical process that begins with adding bacteria, yeast or fungi to food. Any of these will break a food down into its basic components. Along the way, fermentation also acts as a preservative and enhances a food's natural nutrients.

Fermented veggies exhibit a tangy, tart, tingly flavor because of the presence of lactic acid, which essentially evaporates the inherent sugars and carbs in the process. Fermentation creates probiotic, bacteria-building bulwarks restoring balance in your gut, thus aiding your immune system's effectiveness in holding off disease.

Yogurt is famously probiotic with its "active, live cultures," and there are handy, inexpensive yogurt-making machines for the home. But right now, let's look at the fun of ferrying a different fermented food to the finish.

Veggie Fermenting Made Fun

For DIYers, here's how easy it is to create a little culture in your kitchen. Here's what you'll need:

- Vegetable chopper, such as a knife, mandoline slicer or food processor
- Chopping board
- Large bowl or container for the veggies
- Blunt meat pounder or potato masher to brutally, mercilessly pound the liquid content out of inherently juicy vegetables such as cabbage, shredded carrots, etc.
- Unrefined sea salt or pickling salt
- Starter cultures such as whey (a dairy byproduct), kefir grains or commercially produced freeze-dried culture
- Filtered water, for washing the vegetables
- A cylindrical fermenting vessel such as a ceramic crock, wide-mouthed glass jar, slow-cooker insert, glass or ceramic bowl or—if this doesn't sound too repetitive—a specialty ceramic fermenting crock. (Don't use vessels with hard corners or metallic vessels, since they don't play well with salt and fermentation-created acids, and forget plastic containers too; they leech chemicals and are vulnerable to scratches that become hiding places for dangerous bacteria.)
- A weight-and-cover system, depending on what you're fermenting. (Nonbrine fruits, veggies and condiments often don't require weights to keep the food submerged in liquid, but when a brine solution is involved, you'll need a weighting mechanism that fits inside, such as a plate fitting snugly inside the vessel, or a clean rock, smaller jar or other object hefty enough to keep those veggies from sneaking to the surface during their hibernation.)

May the Fermenting *Begin!*

- Scrub the vegetables in filtered water. *Don't* sterilize or cook them— you'll destroy the natural bacteria required during fermentation.
- Slice up all veggies, except any hot peppers you might be using.
- Put the veggies in a big bowl, get out your meat pounder or potato masher and show your produce prey who's boss: pound, squish and commit general mayhem until all the juices are liberated.

- Add salt to taste. Celery juice is a good sodium-free alternative.
- Mix in your starter culture—the whey, kefir grains or freeze-dried culture.
- Got hot peppers? Remove the seeds, chop up the peppers and toss 'em in with their vegetable compatriots.
- Place everything in your glass or ceramic vessel of choice, leaving three inches at the top.
- Push those babies down until the juices come to the top, then weigh the veggies down below the liquid's surface.
- Place a cover atop the vessel, one that keeps bugs out but allows gases to escape and limits oxygen from sneaking in.
- Keep the filled vessel in your kitchen or another warm area. Taste the ferment daily, making sure to keep everything below the liquid-level line. When that telltale tart taste taps you on the tongue, transfer the vessel to the fridge or another cool place for a longer stretch.
- How long is the wait for your fermentin' food to become fabulous? That's often two to twenty-one days, although various factors come into play. The more salt you use, for example, the slower the process. Ditto for cooler room temps. But don't ferment veggies in a very warm room; aim for a reasonable, medium room temperature.
- Generally speaking, once your veggies acquire that tangy taste, they're ready to serve. But while some pickle patrons like their boys soaked for just a week, other gherkin gourmands insist tangier is tastier. They'll submerge theirs up to three weeks in the briny depths. Best bet: Let the taste testing begin a few days in to gauge your personal preference for fermented foodstuffs.

Save It for a Rainy Day

Storing finished, fermented veggies for later use actually can improve their taste. Some home fermenters place vessels in a root cellar or refrigerator for up to six weeks, allowing the flavor to grow fuller naturally. Shelf life varies and can range up to nine months, depending on a ferment's salt content (often 1 to 2 percent). This assumes the fermented veggies are kept in a dark cool location and remain pinned beneath the liquid surface.

Fermented Choices

Fermented foods were around long before the discovery of their restorative power to body defenses. Beyond fermentation's value to the immune system, it also preserves food, enhances nutritional content and makes minerals more easily available for the body to use. Below is some fermented fare to consider, some exotic, others familiar.

- **Veggies.** How's this for a slogan for a national "clean-living" diet campaign? "That some hate veggies is *lamentable*—'cause almost any vegetable is *fermentable*." The most common veggie candidates for culturing include cabbage, cucumbers, carrots, onions, squash, turnips and eggplant. Get creative with fermentation combos such as beets with said carrots or with ginger, garlic, leeks, onions, dulse (seaweed) or jalapeños.
- **Kimchi.** This traditional Korean vegetable side dish is so legendary that it has its own museum in Seoul.[61] Fermented for months in jars buried underground, kimchi (sometimes spelled kimchee) boasts nearly two hundred variations that use as the key ingredient napa cabbage, radishes, scallions, cucumbers and a zillion other veggies.
- **Kombucha.** A carbonated black tea that actually resembles ginger ale, kombucha is the Babe Ruth of fermented drinks because its multitude of microorganisms—including as many as seven probiotic bugs—can do your gut some good.
- **Sauerkraut.** Who knew fermented cabbage, that favorite at delis, diners and hot dog dives, could be such a powerful ally to human

---

61 Perhaps rivaled only by the pioneering (but makeshift) burger museum of American Matt Malmgren, who began collecting McDonald's hamburgers in 1989 and reports they still look exactly the same, even after decades! Where would fast food be without the chemical industry?

health? (If only hot dogs were too.) Besides boosting immunity, 'kraut also helps with brain health and depression, according to Dr. Drew Ramsey, a psychiatrist and the author of books about healthful brain food including *The Happiness Diet* and *50 Shades of Kale.*[62]

- **Pickles.** When you're at the deli pickin' up probiotic-packin' 'kraut, grab some pickles, too. Your friends might think you lack culture, but you'll know better.

- **Coconut yogurt.** This one's recommended by celebrity nutritionist Kimberley Snyder, who appreciates that it's dairy free and chock full of enzymes and probiotics. She prefers it to Greek and regular yogurt, which, while cultured (i.e., fermented), are dairy, acidic and not always easily digested.[63]

- **Miso.** This paste of fermented soybeans and grains is a gold mine of essential minerals and millions of probiotic micro-organisms, according to Jeff Cox, author of *The Essential Book of Fermentation.*[64] No need to scout out Japanese restaurants for miso soup, either. Just plop a dollop of miso paste into boiling water and toss in bok choy, 'shrooms or your favorite vegetables.

- **Tempeh.** Welcome to Protein City. Cox says these fermented whole soybeans, bound into a block-shaped cake during culturing, have all the amino acids you'll need from protein. As such, you can "watch your tempeh" become a nice meat substitute, especially for the bacon in a BLT. Cox also recommends sprinkling tamari— wheat-free soy sauce—onto tempeh before plopping the soy cake onto your newly baconless BLT. Tempeh also enlivens a bowl of steamed veggies.

---

62   Jennifer Kass, *Seven Fermented Foods You Should Be Eating*, Aug. 9, 2013, http://wellandgood. com/2013/08/09/7-fermented-foods-you-should-be-eating/#7-fermented-foods-you-should-be-eating-3.

63   ibid.

64   ibid.

When Probiotic-Treated Pigs Fly?

Here's a little more on probiotics—the so-called "good" or "friendly" bacteria in both food and supplements. For a start, these living organisms—most prominently certain bacteria and yeast—help with digestion. But the overall probiotics picture is much bigger—because they can actually help *prevent* food poisoning altogether by *boosting immunity*. Scientists 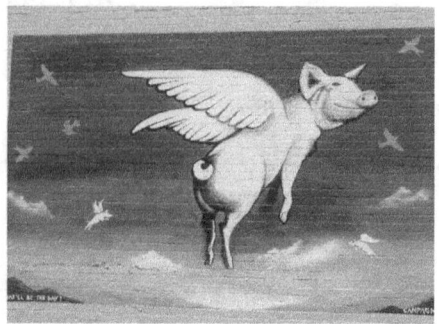 believe they do this by stimulating production of white blood cells, which, in turn, fight off invading hordes of infectious organisms, including those causing food poisoning. Probiotics earn their keep by restoring bacterial balance (and thus overall health) to a large intestine thrown out of whack when harmful bacteria suddenly outnumber good-guy bugs, following either infection, a course of antibiotics or damage to the intestinal lining.

What's important to remember is that you need to take probiotics on a regular and consistent basis for them to work for you.

A 2011 study at Yale University reviewed existing probiotic research and found that besides helping the immune system, probiotics also appear pretty effective in treating these:

- Childhood diarrhea
- Ulcerative colitis
- Necrotizing enterocolitis, an intestinal infection and inflammation affecting infants
- Eczema associated with an allergy to cow's milk

The Yale study also determined probiotics are effective in preventing these conditions:

- Antibiotic-associated diarrhea and infectious diarrhea

- Pouchitis, an inflammation of the intestines that can develop after intestinal surgery

The Yalies also reported encouraging, though hardly definitive, findings that probiotics may also help treat symptoms of irritable bowel syndrome, vaginitis and the infectious diarrhea caused by the bacterium *C. difficile*.

And yet another study in 2010 suggested probiotics might cut the risk of childhood illnesses including ear infections, strep throat and—ta da!—even the common cold.

One last word on probiotics. In an experiment in Ireland, test pigs received probiotic bacteria (five strains of lactic-acid bacteria) in milk and then were infected with salmonella. They fared much better in overall recovery than a control group of pigs receiving plain milk before being infected.

What, you're unimpressed? Not a bacon fan? The study's Irish researchers believe the probiotics' effectiveness may someday be duplicated in humans. "The administered probiotic bacteria improved both the clinical and microbiological outcome of *Salmonella* infection," the researchers reported. "These strains offer significant benefit for use in the food industry and may have potential in human applications." [65]

Pigs today, people tomorrow?

Other Foods to Fine-Tune the System Immune
The following are among the most widely recognized everyday foods that can do a body good:

- ✓ **Yogurt products,** as we've noted earlier, are fermented, semisolid milk and milk solids, with the added bacterial cultures *Lactobacillus bulgaricus* and *Streptococcus thermophiles*. A yogurt cousin, kefir, is fermented cow's milk and, like yogurt, a real pal to the immune system.

---

65 P. G. Casey, G. E. Gardiner, G. Casey, B. Bradshaw, P. G. Lawlor, P. B. Lynch, F. C. Leonard, et al., "A Five-Strain Probiotic Combination Reduces Pathogen Shedding and Alleviates Disease Signs in Pigs Challenged with Salmonella Enterica Serovar Typhimurium," *Applied Environmental Microbiology* 73, no. 6 (2007): 1858–63, http://www.ncbi.nlm.nih.gov/pubmed/17261517.

However, those who have trouble digesting dairy may think twice about yogurt.

✓ **Dark-green leafy vegetables such as spinach, collard greens and kale** contain antioxidants that help fight off eye disorders including cataracts and macular degeneration.

✓ **Cruciferous vegetables to consider include broccoli, cabbage, Brussels sprouts, cauliflower and turnips. These** also boast antioxidants and other nutrients that reduce the risk of cancer.

✓ **Orange and yellow fruits and vegetables like sweet potatoes, carrots, mangoes and apricots** are crammed with carotenoids that heroically shield the immune system.

✓ **Red fruits including tomatoes, watermelon, papaya and pink grapefruit** contain lycopene—not a medication for werewolves but actually a powerful antioxidant combating heart disease and some cancers, particularly that of the prostate. Just don't eat them at midnight during a full moon.

✓ **Blue and purple fruits and vegetables such as blueberries, purple grapes, red cabbage, beets and plums** guard against carcinogens and heart disease.

✓ **Miscellaneous goodies** including garlic, dark chocolate, red wine and black, green and white teas all contain antioxidants. Allegedly.

How All This Helps You

All this Auntie Inflammatory stuff sure *sounds* like the path to improved immunity and clean livin'. But are there *tangible* benefits? You bet:

- **Maintain weight.** Controlling your weight is much easier under this diet.
- **Feel fuller.** Whole foods keep you feeling satisfied longer, thus discouraging the kind of bad snacking you've solemnly sworn to abandon.
- **Regain regularity.** 'Nuff said.

- **Addition by subtraction.** Losing artificial ingredients strengthens your cells and increases the body's efficiency.
- **Slash the risk of disease.** Remember that reducing inflammation goes a long way toward diminishing your chances for heart trouble, cancer, arthritis and other serious illnesses.
- **Micronutrients.** A varied diet of clean foods delivers healthful doses and combinations of essential trace elements, that is, vitamins and minerals, which also reduce cholesterol levels and better regulate blood sugar.
- **Multiply your motivation.** The better you feel, the more you're motivated to take care of yourself in other ways. Okay, maybe this one's not so tangible, but that doesn't make it any less true.

A Review for You

Inflammation didn't start out as humanity's quiet enemy. In fact, it's always been a key part of the body's strategic defenses, helping to spur healing by drawing the body's restorative resources to where they're needed. But in the long-term, low-level inflammation anywhere in the body can destroy one's ability to get and stay healthy. In fact, it's a major source of heart disease, cancer, dementia, rheumatoid arthritis and many other devastating, sometimes fatal illnesses.

One of the best and tastiest ways to fight inflammation is through diet, especially a "clean" (i.e., anti-inflammatory) strategy based on probiotics-rich whole (i.e., natural) foods that haven't emerged from a manufacturing plant ground, reformed, processed, reconstituted, refined, altered, preserved, hypnotized, bastardized or otherwise transformed into something *unholy* by smirking little men in white lab coats.

One easy way to deliver probiotics to your dinner table is through the joy of fermented foods. It's even fun to make them yourself.

And then there are the many herbs and spices that bring great, varied flavors to clean livin' meals, not to mention the crucial vitamins and nutrients that just might become life savers for you and those you love.

"What You Can Do" Checklist: 'Tis the Seasoning—A Shopping List

One way to jump-start a stalled or compromised immune system is revealed in the paraphrasing of a landmark folk song: "To every thing, there is a seasoning."[66] You really can sprinkle your way to a better place, immunologically speaking—and do so *sans salt*.

Besides, adding sodium chloride for taste is what's gotten too many in trouble—regardless of whether you salted it yourself, passively acquired it in a fast food burger, or gobbled down snack crackers and other processed "food."

Instead, there are a gazillion other spices and herbs out there—healthful sprinkables without the threatening properties of sodium. The following things help with heart health, can reduce inflammation and can even challenge cancer. Oh yeah, they add panache to mealtimes too:

✓ **Cinnamon.** Good old cinnamon is one powerful anti-inflammatory and antioxidant, shielding cells from oxidative stress and the threats of free radicals,[67] Alzheimer's, diabetes, Parkinson's, cancer and cardiovascular issues. It also lowers levels of blood sugar, heart-cloggin' LDL ("bad") cholesterol and triglycerides. Plus, a compound in cinnamon prevents blood platelets from clumping unnecessarily. Cinnamon oil may actually become a factor in preventing *E. coli* infections. A study at Washington State University found the oil can be a very effective, natural antibacterial agent with potential applications in food manufacturing and processing. The ultimate result could be stopping *E. coli* cases before they begin.[68] Try cinnamon on fresh fruit, desserts,

---

66 "Turn, Turn, Turn (To Everything There Is a Season)," by Pete Seeger, lyrics from Ecclesiastes 3:1–8 (Authorized Version).

67 Not a college activist from the 1960s. Actually, a free radical is a perfectly reasonable molecule that, having lost a critical electron (don't ask why), pulls a Jekyll/Hyde and goes on a maniacal, wild-eyed reign of terror in search of the replacement electron it needs ~~for world conquest~~ to be a stable, upright member of proper molecular society. Under the right conditions in the body, free radicals can multiply exponentially, causing a chain reaction of cell carnage in the body. Without the presence of sufficient antioxidants, often from vitamins C and E, you're in big trouble.

68 Lina Sheng, Mei-Jun Zhu, "Inhibitory Effect of Cinnamomum cassia Oil on Non-O157 Shiga Toxin-Producing Escherichia coli," *Food Control* 46 (Dec. 2014): 374-381.

curries, in coffee and tea, in oatmeal, with a scoop of peanut butter or on fish, chicken or lamb. You can even combine cinnamon with cumin and chili powder for a Middle Eastern touch to meat dishes. But beware—the vast majority of "cinnamon" sold in the United States is actually a cousin called cassia. Real cinnamon, usually labeled "Ceylon cinnamon," is derived from the bark of a tree native to Sri Lanka, the island nation once known as Ceylon. Most cinnamon in the United States is labeled "canela molida," simply Spanish for...cinnamon. However, real cinnamon has higher levels of antioxidants, so it's worth scouting around for the real deal.

✓ **Basil.** With a leaf roughly the color of lime Jell-O, this flavorful herb is filled with flavonoids for antioxidant protection, plenty of potassium for building muscle, manganese for bone formation, vitamin A for improved immunity, vision and cell growth and vitamin K for healthy bones and other benefits. The best known among more than sixty varieties is sweet basil, famously used in Italian food and the star attraction in pesto sauce. Among other varieties, lemon and Thai basils are associated with Asian dishes. And holy basil[69] (also known as either tulsi or pepper basil) is related to sweet basil but with a clove flavor far afield from the sweet stuff. Basil is a great last-second addition to healthful stir-fries, especially those with eggplant, cabbage, chili peppers, tofu and cashew nuts. Other candidates for recipe basilization[70] are tomato sauces, dressings and spreads, soup, and beef, pork, chicken and fish. You can even brew basil tea by boiling chopped basil leaves in water for eight minutes. Spiritually minded gourmands know that holy basil is worshiped by Hindus as the incarnation of the wife of Vishnu, their faith's main deity.[71]

✓ **Marjoram.** Often confused with its close cousin oregano, this aromatic herb's chemical makeup has anti-inflammatory powers far beyond

---

69 Not affiliated with Batman's crime-fighting partner Robin or any other known superhero.

70 No such word exists. You read it here first. Patent pending®.

71 No kidding. This is true. Honest. You could look it up.

those of mortal men. Marjoram spices up veggies including peas,[72] spinach, tomatoes and carrots. It also plays nice with stews, soup and beef, although we don't advocate beefing up your meat intake just for the sake of marjoram.

✓ **Mint.** More than just a kicky flavor for candy, gum and breath fresheners, this plant's serious side inspired this bumper sticker idea: "Real Mint Fights Cancer." Perillyl alcohol, a chemical in mint, draws a line in the sand for invading cancer cells. Add to that mint's generous endowment of beta-carotene, heart-healthy folate and riboflavin, the last of these fulfilling your recommended daily allowance (RDA) of riboes.[73] Besides desserts, mint works well on both fruit and leafy salads, as a garnish for pudding, or in tea.

✓ **Oregano.** *Don't call it marjoram!* Sensitive, prideful oregano loves its botanic cousin but prefers to stand on its own record of healthful nutrients including iron, fiber, calcium, vitamins C and A and omega-3 fatty acids. Sprinkle this sexy antioxidant herb into a potful of homemade red sauce with reckless abandon. Don't stop there—dressings, salads (especially Greek), soups, sauces, gravies and meat dishes—chicken, fish and pork—all scream for oregano.

✓ **Parsley.** That ubiquitous parsley garnish atop restaurant entrées is useless. Purely for cosmetic purposes, right? Wrong! The innocent-looking little sprig boasts healthful doses of vitamin C, iron, calcium and potassium. Its flavonoids are strong antioxidants and its folate content guards against heart disease. Sneak parsley into salads and rice pilaf, onto grilled fish and into sauces and gravies.

✓ **Sage.** A wise person knows sage is a favorite of Auntie Inflammatory and her first cousin, Auntie Oxidants. This learned herb helps with memory, mood and digestion. It's also a sworn enemy of Alzheimer's and other dementia disorders. Sage knows its way around comfort food like casseroles and adds flavor to roasted sweet potatoes,

---

72 Okay, okay, it's a legume, we know.

73 A complete fiction. There's no such thing as a ribo. But riboflavin, an alias for vitamin B_2, is not only quite real but also vital to metabolizing energy and powering many body processes on the cellular level.

butternut squash soup, red sauces, soups, stews and the eggs-quisite frittata and its utterly whipped cousin, the omelet. And to every season, there is an herb—for sage, autumn is the time when it enlivens both turkey stuffing and the bird itself.

✓ **Rosemary.** Don't let the pretty name fool you—this rosemary is one tough cookie, standing up to those devilish free radicals, to inflammation and also to estrogens linked to breast cancer. Chopped and sprinkled, this aromatic herb adds flavor to soups, stews, lamb, beef and chicken. Want a healthful dip but your hot tub is in dry dock? Try rosemary in olive oil for an elegant dip ideal with warm, hearty whole-grain sprouted bread. And here's a favorite that never gets old: Wrap smoked-salmon slices around asparagus stalks. Sprinkle with olive oil and rosemary, then bake at 375 degrees Fahrenheit for about ten minutes. This fabulous finger food makes a great appetizer and low-carb snack.

✓ **Thyme.** This minty/lemony-tasting aromatic herb is almost supernaturally powerful in promoting good health. A 2004 study showed its oil extract, thymol, is so antimicrobial that it actually decontaminated lettuce infected with the nasty food poison shigella.[74] Clean-livin' thymol also is used in mouthwashes and some green-colored household cleaning liquids. Medically speaking, thyme is found to combat staph and *E. coli*, help digestion, reduce gas and, for the follicularly fixated, benefit the hair and scalp. As a food flavoring, thyme goes well with root vegetables, egg dishes, chicken and fish, especially salmon, where lemon and thyme pool their tasty resources to produce a swimmingly delicious entrée.

✓ **Tarragon.** Licorice lovers will take to tarragon; they taste similar, although tarragon is just a tad sweeter. Health-wise, tarragon slashes the overboard stickiness of blood platelets and is loaded with beta-carotene and potassium. This herb is on great terms with both chicken

---

74   C. F. Bagamboula, M. Uyttendaele and J. Debevere, "Inhibitory Effect of Thyme and Basil Essential Oils, Carvacrol, Thymol, Estragol, Linalool and p-cymene toward *Shigella sonnei* and *S. flexneri*," *Food Microbiology* 21, no. 1 (2004): 33–42.

and fish, can moonlight as a salad green, is a taste maker in dressing and loves to mix it up with Greek-yogurt appetizer dips.

✓ **Cloves.** These dried, pink, handpicked, nutrient-rich, unopened buds of the evergreen clove tree contain manganese, omega-3 fatty acids but *especially* a ton of the yellow-colored oil eugenol.[75] This multitasking oil is truly a Renaissance chemical compound, fighting not just joint inflammation but also listeria and digestive-tract cancers. Eugenol also is believed to prevent toxicity from environmental pollutants. It even gets a workout in dentistry as a mild anesthetic and antibacterial agent. Cloves' sweet, fragrant taste has been featured in Asian cuisines for two millennia. And back in the day, it was even used to freshen breath. For cooking, cloves should be pulverized into powder with a coffee grinder before being sprinkled into soups, broths, hot tea, coffee, stuffing and after-dinner treats including fruit compote and apple desserts.

✓ **Cumin.** This antioxidant seed is derived from a flowering plant native to a wide area from the eastern Mediterranean to India. Cumin is a spice that cuts cancer risk and contains immune-boosting metals including iron and manganese. Cumin is great in chili, Tex-Mex recipes, stir-fry veggies, Middle Eastern dishes and rice pilaf. And don't let this get around, but when combined with black pepper and honey, cumin is considered an aphrodisiac in some Middle Eastern countries. This is purely for informational purposes, so don't get any ideas.

✓ **Nutmeg.** This warmly pungent spice is naturally loaded with vital nutrients that lower blood pressure and boast antioxidant and antifungal properties. Keep whole nutmegs, which resemble acorns, in an airtight container, and with a nutmeg grater (or little rasp[76]), grind up a fresh supply just before use. Don't grate and store ahead of time because nutmeg quickly loses the oils behind its flavor and taste. Nutmeg adds a nice touch to hot tea and curry powder and a thrill to such diverse dishes as baked ziti, apricot-date chutney and banana

---

75 Other good sources of eugenol include cinnamon, basil, bay leaf and nutmeg.
76 For a bigger rasp, Rod Stewart's music is available via download and CD.

muffins, and it is very kind to desserts including the beloved pudding brothers, rice and bread.

✓ **Saffron.** This concentrated, classic flavoring has the distinction of being the most expensive spice on earth, going for $1,500 per pound and up. Luckily, saffron's usually sold by the gram, which brings the price down to under fifteen dollars for a supply that can last months. As little as a tenth of a teaspoon can also help as an antidepressant. And by increasing blood flow to the brain, saffron helps heighten cognitive performance. In the kitchen, it brings magic to paella, risotto and other rice dishes; saffron is a great accent on garlic-herb chicken and many other chicken dishes; and it's a flavorful spike in bouillabaisse and other specialty recipes.

✓ **Turmeric.** Why in the world would you care about a spice that blocks cancer from spreading and is a valuable anti-inflammatory—a spice that protects the cardiovascular system, slows down Alzheimer's disease, helps control weight, may be an effective painkiller (especially for osteoarthritis) and is an antiseptic? You'd be *insane* to turn to turmeric and its powerful, multitasking phytochemical, curcumin. Seriously, why ever would you want a spice that's a low-cost alternative to saffron and so healthful it even makes an excellent tea—one that goes well with sauces, Indian food, lentil soup, egg salad, fish recipes and chicken dishes, among others? *Why? Why? Why?*

✓ **Ginger.** This zingy spice—neither sweet nor bitter, but intriguingly in-between—could stand alone as a versatile, effective over-the-counter treatment for nausea, as an insurance policy against gastric ulcers, as a digestion aid and as a pain mitigator for menstrual cramps, muscle discomfort, migraines, osteoarthritis and other forms of chronic inflammation. But be careful: For some, taking large dietary doses of ginger can bring heartburn and gas, worsen gallstones or spur unwanted drug interactions, particularly with warfarin, the anticoagulant medication used by heart patients.[77] So check with your doctor before jammin' with ginger. If you

---

77 Warfarin may be better known by brand names including Coumadin, Jantoven, Marevan and Uniwarfin.

get the go-ahead, ginger is a good thing to go with daily. But find fresh ginger, not the powdered stuff. If your supermarket disappoints, try an Asian market—ginger's a staple in Asian and Indian cuisines. Ginger is terrific in baked goods, most famously gingerbread and gingersnaps but also muffins, cakes and many other desserts.

✓ **Chili peppers.** Last, but decidedly not least, we present the mighty chili pepper. Neither herb nor spice, the pepper is actually a fruit (not a veggie) and boasts a trademark pungency (i.e., hotness) that makes you sweaty, teary-eyed and famously flush from what feels like a fleeting food fever. A pepper's pungency reflects its level of capsaicin, an antioxidant chemical compound that stimulates chemical receptor nerve endings in the skin. Not coincidentally, the more capsaicin in a pepper, the greater its antioxidant power. Peppers also contain vitamins and nutrients that help reduce the risks of breast and ovarian cancer, preserve eyesight, assist the body's natural chemical processes and help brain and immune functions. Peppers also are believed to be modest appetite suppressors. Plus, these little hotties release endorphins—pain-control biochemicals also appreciated as mankind's "pleasure hormones." (No wonder the ancient Aztecs and Mayans considered peppers an aphrodisiac.[78]) Habaneros, among the hottest of the hot, have the most capsaicin; jalapeños have some, green peppers, predictably, none at all. Over time and repeated exposure, the tender tongues of pepper neophytes become desensitized to the spicy pain—making peppers even more satisfying in meals. For some people, peppers are like raw oysters, haggis and martial arts films—an acquired taste. So beginners should start with blander varieties and remove the veins and seeds, which are the hottest parts. In cooking, peppers are good for spiking up marinades, sauces, salsas and guacamole; in breakfast egg dishes (remember: organic eggs whenever possible); on fish including salmon, tilapia and halibut; with shellfish[79]

---

78 Any gifted chef armed with a recipe featuring both (alleged) aphrodisiacs cumin and chili peppers could rule the world.

79 Be sure you're not allergic, since for some people shellfish can be delicious but deadly.

including sautéed shrimp, scallops and lobster; on chicken; and with countless other foods.

When You're Hot, You're Hot: Charting Chili Peppers

Mild chili peppers	Medium-hot chili peppers	*Call an ambulance!*
Sweet peppers: • Green • Yellow genetics • Red chili Chili verde Anaheim Pablano Pasilla Chilaca	Guajillo Jalapeño Yellow hot	Serrano Manzano Arbol Cayenne Habanero

When No Food Is Good Food

Want to boost your immune system and slash your grocery bill at the same time? Then try putting this on your dinner plate:

Nothing.

In June 2014, researchers at the University of Southern California found that fasting for four to five days will actually trigger stem cell–based regeneration of the immune system. In short, you can rebuild your immune system by not eating.

USC researcher Valter Longo told *The Daily Beast* that holding to a fast diet ranging from 750 to 1,050 calories a day for at least four to five days will do the trick. And he said humans can follow the diet every one to three months.

The study reported the depletion of white blood cells during these fasts is what gives the immune system its renewed vigor.

The findings offer hope for people in particular need of strong immune systems—especially cancer patients facing chemotherapy and people with aging issues. The USC study found fasting may also help extend human longevity.

Not a bad tradeoff for going a little hungry every now and then.

Afterword: Not One and Done

Have we covered a lot of ground *or what?* Let's celebrate with a little stocktaking. In ten glorious chapters, we

- Surveyed food warnings and recalls ranging from the common to the just plain weird;[80]
- Educated you on the nastiest microbial miscreants and food-borne pathogens;
- Provided best practices on safely shopping, storing and preparing food;
- Offered priceless advice on eating safely in restaurants, at fairs, from food trucks, while traveling and at the holidays;[81]
- Revealed the potential perils and pitfalls posed by pet food;
- Demystified the world of food dating—no, not cozy dinners with that cute number cruncher from accounting; actually, we addressed the naked truths about expiration, fresh-until and use-by dates;
- Recommended simple treatments, should microbial monsters have their way with you;

---

80 Don't say you've already forgotten Wisconsin's own snackin' Emma Schweiger, who retrieved from the depths of her bag of chips a cell phone. Still no word on roaming charges.
81 With a tip 'o' the hat to good old Uncle Phil Shear, 1932–2012. Miss you, Phil.

- Shared the essence of the clean-living (anti-inflammatory) diet;
- And finally, offered up a megaselection of food choices and alternatives to keep your body in balance and hold microbial mayhem at bay.

But one final, important point remains. Let's go for the dramatic setup:

You're doubled over, the twisted expression on your face underscoring the agony in your gut. Plus, is that a fever or are we inside a blast furnace?

Before you know it, your lunch is making a sudden and surprise comeback in one of two ways, neither requiring elaboration.

Is this the cosmic payoff for a weekend of binge viewing *Here Comes Honey Boo Boo*? Maybe. But mostly, your symptoms provide ugly yet unmistakable evidence of "food poisoning," the umbrella term for any number of dangerous food-borne bacteria.

"Ah, just a stomach bug," you reassure the family. "Probably just a twenty-four-hour thing."

Better hope that's all it is.

Better yet, pay attention and don't summarily shrug off symptoms as merely the tame, temporary toxicity of tainted food. Because what you've got could be not only dangerous but long-term and even life-threatening.

We Spell Danger "C-O-M-P-L-I-C-A-T-I-O-N-S"

Among the consequences of food-borne illnesses we've discussed, dehydration is the most common. Drinking water and other clear fluids provides a pretty easy fix. If only other bacterial complications were so easy to smack down. As we noted in chapter 1, food-borne illness can lead to devastating conditions including the hemolytic-uremic and Guillain-Barré syndromes, reactive arthritis and postinfectious irritable bowel syndrome.

So take your gastrointestinal illness seriously—because many of these infections can take your life altogether or make it needlessly and painfully complicated for years to come.

A Final Word

So now you know just how (unfortunately) easy it is to acquire food-borne illness and potential complications. You also have at your fingertips powerful information, simple food strategies and commonsense caution to keep yourself and loved ones safe from all methods of microbial madness. Plus, you're armed with the basics of Auntie Inflammatory's clean-living diet, allowing you to blaze a new path across your kitchen linoleum toward a safer, healthier and arguably tastier life.

As such, you owe us, the authors, big time. No worries—we ask just one simple favor: *don't shove this volume onto some bookshelf and forget about it.* Don't let this become just another anonymous, vaguely remembered title lost in a sea of neglected cookbooks, self-help manuals and cheesy pop-lit novels. Instead, keep it within easy reach in the kitchen. Refer to it often. Keep the concepts and suggestions in these pages alive and part of your daily routine. Tell your family and friends what you've learned.

Without proselytizing, of course. That's our job.

And don't stress! Maybe you're wondering, "What if I fall off the wagon and break rules I learned here?" Simple answer:

So what? "Tomorrow," as a certain fictional heroine once noted, "is another day."[82]

Cut yourself slack and begin anew the next day with fresh resolve—and basil—to cook and dine well and generally regard food as among the best opportunities for you to take control of your own life and health.

Which leads to our final movie quote, from Ruth Gordon as Maude, a zesty, seventy-nine-year-old, life-affirming concentration camp survivor:

"Go team, *go!* Give me an L! Give me an I! Give me a V! Give me an E! L-I-V-E. *Live!* Otherwise…you got nothin' to talk about in the locker room."[83]

Or, for that matter, in the kitchen.

---

82 Our penultimate movie reference is the final line of 1939's *Gone with the Wind*, delivered by Vivien Leigh in her Academy Award®-winning role as Scarlett O'Hara.

83 *Harold and Maude*, 1971, original screenplay by Colin Higgins. You should own a copy of this film. Especially if you're curious about organic wine and oat-straw tea.

www.ingramcontent.com/pod-product-compliance
Lightning Source LLC
Chambersburg PA
CBHW071359280526
45787CB00001B/380